KEYS TO UNDERSTANDING OSTEOPOROSIS

Jan Rozek, R.N.

BARRON'S

Medical illustrations by Lillian Michael
Exercise drawings by Catherine Blaski Liptack

Copyright © 1992 by Barron's Educational Series, Inc.

All inquiries should be addressed to:
Barron's Educational Series, Inc.
250 Wireless Boulevard
Hauppauge, New York 11788

Library of Congress Catalog Card No. 91-41280

International Standard Book No. 0-8120-4664-1

Library of Congress Cataloging in Publication Data

Rozek, Jan.
    Keys to understanding osteoporosis / Jan Rozek.
        p.   cm.—(Barron's retirement keys)
    Includes index.
    ISBN 0-8120-4664-1
    1. Osteoporosis—Popular works.   I. Title.   II. Series.
RC931.073R68   1992
616.7'16—dc20   91-41280
                                                                    CIP

PRINTED IN THE UNITED STATES OF AMERICA
2345   5500   987654321

1

CONTENTS

DEDICATION

I would like to dedicate this book to my husband, Ray, my wellspring of support, who challenges me to achieve beyond my dreams.

To our three daughters, Terry, Lisa, and Maria, our blessings, our joy, our future.

And to all the young people whose health we, as adults, have an obligation to safeguard.

To Aunt Agnes Hahm, lively and loving role model for all of us, in celebration of over ninety years of successful living.

In memory of my parents, Ben and Martha Goecks, source of my life's values, and our son, Michael.

And to Emily.

ACKNOWLEDGMENTS

I wish to express my sincere appreciation to those who enriched this book with their exceptional expertise. I am grateful to Charles R. Wilson, Ph.D., associate professor of radiology, Medical College of Wisconsin, Milwaukee, for assistance and review of the Keys on densitometry; Stephen Machinton, M.D., S.C., attending staff, Department of Obstetrics and Gynecology, Columbia Hospital, Milwaukee, Wisconsin, for review of the Keys on postmenopausal osteoporosis and hormone replacement therapy; Frank J. Bonner, M.D., chairman, Department of Physical Medicine and Rehabilitation, The Graduate Hospital, Philadelphia, Pennsylvania, for information for the Keys on rehabilitation and physical comfort measures; Jean A. Kahl, P.T., for assistance and review of the Keys on exercise and fractures; and Cathy Blaski-Liptack for drawings for the Key on exercise.

I wish to thank personnel at the National Osteoporosis Foundation and National Institutes of Health for graciously providing helpful resources. I am indebted to David W. Dempster, Ph.D., director, Regional Bone Center, Helen Hayes Hospital, and associate professor for clinical pathology, Columbia University, New York, for reviewing the entire manuscript to assure accuracy. His valuable suggestions have been incorporated into the text.

I am also deeply grateful for the vote of confidence of Allison St. Claire, senior wire, and for the encouragement and good counsel of my friend, Doris Jean Rand, and members of my support group, Laura De Nooyer-Moore, Steve Lowry, Elizabeth Martorell, Maynard McKillen, Tom Meyer, Myron Ratkowski, and Mary Sather.

With special appreciation to scientists, researchers, physicians, and all others involved in health care, whose efforts enable the thread of optimism that is woven through the fabric of this book; to those who, by reading it, express their will to live more healthfully; and to Carolyn Horne, my editor at Barron's, whose proficiency and forbearance made this book possible.

INTRODUCTION

When I was ten years old, a friend of our family came to visit . I believe she changed my life. She was hunched over, her shoulders stooped. Her long white hair was twisted into a bun snuggled against the back of her neck. Balancing on two canes, Emily charmed me with stories of her childhood, recalling playing tag and climbing trees. She strained to look up at me from her bent position. Later I learned the cause of Emily's tragic posture.

"It comes from not drinking enough milk," my mother told me.

I was stunned. For as long as I could remember, I'd disliked milk and refused to drink it. Until I met Emily. Today, I know that milk is only part of the complex story of osteoporosis.

Perhaps the posture your mother encouraged in your youth, with reminders to "Stand up straight," is yielding to stooped shoulders. Osteoporosis already may be your silent companion, threatening a broken bone with the smallest misstep or unexpected movement. Clothing in your wardrobe may seem longer, when what really is happening is that you are getting shorter, due to fractures of vertebrae.

Perhaps you have stepped from a curb, or moved your arm to brace yourself and painfully discovered how fragile your bones are. A fracture may, in fact, have opened the door, introduced you to osteoporosis, and invited the first step of a treatment program. Maybe your bones are strong and healthy; you will want to keep them that way. Whatever your circumstance, decide today to learn about osteoporosis so you can take proper care of yourself.

If you understand the benefits of lifestyle changes that you need to make, you will be eager to make them and be more fully committed. You can avoid or reduce the following:

- Fractures and their life-threatening complications
- Chronic problems, such as pain, deformity, difficult breathing, disability
- Depression that often accompanies long-term illness and dependency
- Social withdrawal and isolation
- Nursing home placement

With simple lifestyle changes, you are more likely to:

- Look and feel better
- Have a positive outlook on life and a good self-image
- Stay independent, active, and productive.
- Live longer and enjoy improved quality and richness of life

Knowledge is power. And armed power is essential. Weapons include education, proper diet, regular exercise, positive lifestyle habits, early diagnosis, treatment as necessary, and medically directed self-management. Because you are taking the responsibility to find out about osteoporosis, what is involved in prevention and treatment, and what you can do to achieve the best condition possible, you can take a prominent role in your own health management, confident in your ability to make informed decisions. You are in charge.

A physician's highest calling historically has been to heal disease. The modern physician, trained in the value of prevention, still primarily views medicine from a healing perspective. No one has more to gain from pursuing the highest level of fitness, harmony, and well-being than you do. Your doctors and other health providers—dieticians, nurses, pharmacists, and therapists—will advise and assist you, and based on the best information available, help *you* decide what *you* will do. *You* follow through. And *you* reap the benefits.

If you lead a full and active life, it is hard to picture yourself as disabled unless you meet an Emily, or are otherwise forewarned of the danger of osteoporosis. As life spans lengthen, the risks grow. Whether you are nineteen or ninety, good health is your dearest treasure. Guard it with your life.

1

OSTEOPOROSIS: AN EPIDEMIC

Cholera, smallpox, influenza, osteoporosis. Osteoporosis? If you were likely to be struck down by an epidemic, wouldn't you at least know its name? More than 25 million Americans, most of them women, are victims of osteoporosis. By age sixty-five, one of three women will experience an osteoporotic fracture. Men succumb later in life. Estimates project that in less than ten years, 40 percent of our population will live to be eighty-five years old, rendering men equally susceptible.

Postmenopausal women, no longer protected by estrogen, are at greatest risk. Nine out of ten women age seventy-five and older have some degree of osteoporosis. By age eighty, women may lose up to two thirds of their total *bone mass* or tissue. At the turn of the last century, women did not live long enough to experience menopause. By the turn of the next century, women will spend at least one third of their lives in the postmenopausal period!

Osteoporosis. The word defines itself. "Osteo" means bone, and "porosis" refers to the porous structure that results from the gradual loss of bone mass. Osteoporosis is a complicated disease with many interacting elements. Knowledge of cause and treatment is incomplete, making it one of the most common, yet least understood, diseases of middle and old age. Its insidious, unchecked march leaves bones fragile and weak and easily broken. Some experts believe that osteoporosis has reached epidemic proportions among older Americans. The National Institutes of Health lists it as a leading cause of death among older women after heart disease, cancer, and stroke. Yet many victims are unfamiliar with the name and less than 10 percent consider it life threatening. It is especially alarming

1

that many are unmotivated or unequipped to halt its devastating advance.

The tragedy of osteoporosis is due to fractures—1.3 million a year—causing pain, disability, deformity, and death. Common fracture sites are the wrists, hips, and bones of the spine (*vertebrae*). Unless a drastic reversal is effected—and this can be done—33 percent of elderly women and 17 percent of elderly men will suffer hip fractures due to osteoporosis. Hip fractures are a leading cause of lost independence, a catastrophic event, especially for the aged. Twenty percent of these patients will be confined to a wheelchair within a year and 20 percent will need nursing home placement. Nearly one third of the women living in nursing homes are there because of fractures, 85 percent of them fractures of the hip. Twenty percent of those who sustain hip fractures will die within one year as a result.

This grim picture is changing, largely due to a changing attitude. No longer willing to passively receive medical treatment, individuals are more vigilant regarding their health, even anxious to be actively involved. As the media alerts us to the dangers of osteoporosis, men and women are responding in growing numbers, requesting information and advice. Health care providers are finally addressing the issue more aggressively. Many hospitals and clinics now offer patient and community education programs to help individuals assess their risk for developing osteoporosis. They design a prevention plan, provide treatment as necessary, and monitor progress. Increased interest is paying off in individual moves toward prevention, diagnosis, and treatment.

Expense is a sobering issue. The cost of treatment and care is estimated to be $10 billion a year and growing, along with public concern. The cost is expected to triple in the next 30 years, according to the National Osteoporosis Foundation. The human cost is immeasureable—and unacceptable.

Research on this complex health problem has been greatly expanded, another benefit of heightened awareness. Science has made encouraging breakthroughs in a broad spectrum of areas, yielding improved methods to protect our skeleton. New therapies and tests are improving diagnosis and treatment.

The challenge is to inform the public of the latest information about osteoporosis. Educational efforts must be expanded to persuade and assist individuals to build and maintain their bones to the highest level of health. Seeds of hope are coming from ongoing research. The promise of controlling osteoporosis is alive and growing. An informed public, applying the knowledge of medical research, will reduce the widespread incidence of osteoporosis and perhaps one day cause its demise.

This book will furnish information, guidance, and incentive to help you embrace a "wellness" lifestyle. Inform your children and grandchildren, friends, relatives, and neighbors of the compelling message: *osteoporosis is preventable and treatable*. Pass it on! If you convince even one other person to practice prevention, it could save that person's life. What greater gift for those you love than the gift of health?

2

THE STORY OF BONES

From the earliest times, the human skeleton has been considered a mystery and a miracle. Scientific examination was forbidden for centuries by church and state. In A.D. 200, Galen, physician to the Roman emperor Marcus Aurelius, was the first anatomist of the ancient world. Although his teachings, based on animal studies, were false, Galen's writings served as a medical text until the mid-sixteenth century. In 1536, a Belgian physician, Andreas Vesalius, studying human bones stolen from the gallows in Louvain, corrected Galen's work, and anatomy was reborn, based on fact.

While anatomists perfected scientific data, painters, sculptors, and writers of the Renaissance remolded society's regard for the human body by hailing its beauty and vitality, lifting the veil of taboos and religious restrictions. The human form, anatomically and exquisitely correct, disrobed, and stepped into the light to be scrutinized, sparking interest and examination and producing knowledge.

In the next two centuries, more intricacies of bones were revealed. The treatment of disease and deformity of the skeleton became a medical specialty called *orthopaedia*, from the Greek word "orthos," which means straight, free from deformity, and "paidios," a child. The invention of the microscope enabled doctors to study the structure and formation of bone cells.

In 1896, Wilhelm Roentgen discovered X rays, enabling physicians to view the once hidden cracks and crevices, growths and deformities of bones. Since that time, research and knowledge have flourished, unmasked by technology. Bones, once thought to be lifeless and still, proved to be living and dynamic: moving, growing, mending, modeling, and remodeling, every moment, day and night.

From the first hint of life forming in the womb until the day they return to dust, our bones are continually changing. Whereas the adult skeleton has 206 bones, infants are born with about 275, mainly cartilage, like the cusps of our ears and the soft, flexible tips of our noses. Cartilage is gradually replaced by bone tissue, which hardens with mineral deposits, a slow process called *mineralization*, or *calcification*. In short bones, like those in our wrists and ankles, the hardening process begins at the center and moves outward. Long bones in our arms and legs start to change both in the middle and ends, and harden from both directions. Flat bones, like those in our ribs, form from membranes. They become hard on the surface, but remain spongy bone inside.

As we grow older, other changes occur. Bones grow in diameter as layers of bone are added around the outside and removed from the inside of the shaft. Thus the compact bone does not get thicker but the marrow cavity gets larger. Some bones grow together. For example, the nine separate bones at the lower end of the spine fuse into two, the sacrum and coccyx. Our spine, relatively straight at birth, develops curves that help us balance in an upright position with the least possible strain as we begin to hold our heads up, sit, and stand.

The size, shape, and composition of different bones depends on their function. Fingers are fashioned to grasp the tiniest objects. Women have a broader pelvis to yield to childbirth. In addition, different parts of our bodies have different growth patterns. The skull grows rapidly, reaching its full size by age six. Limbs grow faster later. And cell by cell, inch by inch, our bones grow longer, wider, harder, denser, and stronger.

The story of bones, like bones themselves, is anything but dry. (Depending on the type, about one fourth of bone is water.) Let's learn more.

3

HOW YOUR BONES ARE MADE

Skeletal bones form the framework of your body, giving it shape, providing support and stability, and sheltering and protecting the organs and tissues within. Bones serve as connecting points for muscles and tendons, enabling mobility, function, and activity. In addition to their mechanical function, bones are storehouses for minerals, particularly bone-building calcium. Finally, blood cells are manufactured in bone marrow, which is hidden deep within bone.

Two types of bone tissue, *cortical* and *trabecular,* exist. The proportion of each type depends on the particular bone. Cortical (compact) bone forms the hard outer shell. It is very dense, with no open spaces except for tiny channels that serve as passageways for nerves and for the blood vessels that aid bone *metabolism.* Metabolism is the process whereby cells receive nutrients and oxygen and excrete waste products as bone is built up and broken down. Cortical bone forms the shaft of long bones. It composes about 80 percent of the body's total bone.

The inner, cancellous bone is made of a lacy network of marrow-filled spaces separated by thin processes of bone called trabeculae. It is nourished by the soft marrow that fills its hollow cavities and produces blood cells. Sponge-like in appearance, the honeycombed ends of long bones and the bodies of the vertebrae contain trabecular bone. Except at joints, bones are covered by a tough fibrous membrane, the *periosteum.* It is richly supplied with nerves and blood vessels that branch into the bone for nourishment. It also contains cells for bone building and repair.

Bone is 70 percent mineral by weight. The rest is organic material: bone cells, blood and blood vessels, fats, and *collagen,* 95 percent, a tough protein that is woven into tissue fibers. It is the combination of minerals and collagen in the bone *matrix* that gives bones their hardness, flexibility, and strength.

A familiar form of the organic protein of bone (collagen) is gelatin. When boiled in water, collagen yields gelatin. It is gelatin that collects on top of the broth when homemade chicken soup cools. Gelatin in meats, desserts, ice cream, and baked goods is made in a similar manner.

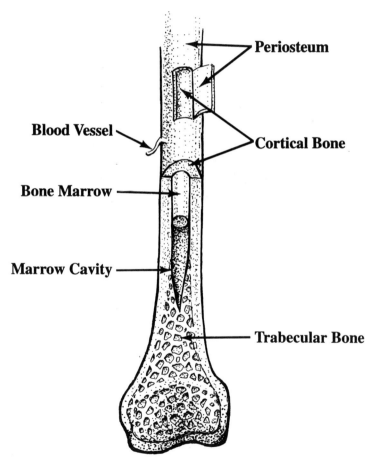

Lower Femur

To observe the hardening quality of the inorganic substance of bone (minerals), place a long bone of a chicken in a jar and cover it with vinegar. Wait a week, then add fresh vinegar. Examine the bone and you will notice that it becomes flexible as minerals are leached out. This is an excellent visual aid to impress children and grandchildren of their body's need for calcium.

The process of making bone is similar to making honey. Bees produce a substance, which they shape into a honeycomb, then gather nectar from flowers to line the spaces in the honeycomb. Similarly, bone cells produce collagen fibers, which they wind and twist into a honeycomb, then gather mineral crystals from the bloodstream to line the spaces in the matrix.

There are three kinds of bone cells: osteoclasts, osteoblasts, and osteocytes. Osteoclasts and osteoblasts work together in bone construction crews, precisely programmed at the local level and also by systemic control of hormones from the endocrine glands. *Osteoclasts* are the demolition cells. They appear at a specified site and, over a period of several weeks, secrete collagen-splitting enzymes and mineral-dissolving acids that burrow holes the size of a pinhead and break down the bony matrix, releasing calcium into the bloodstream.

Osteoblasts are the builders. When osteoclasts have finished their work, osteoblasts from the periosteum move in to form and deposit new tissue. Osteoblasts first manufacture collagen, as well as a cement-like substance in which the collagen fibers are embedded. Next mineral crystals are deposited, completing the matrix. Layer after layer of fresh bone is put down over a period of several months, filling in the tunnels dug by osteoclasts and creating new structural units of bone.

The process whereby old bone is dissolved *(resorption)* and new bone formed is called *remodeling*. Usually the two processes are coupled so that resorption and formation take place at the same rate. Under some circumstances remodeling results in a slight loss of bone, with the total skeletal loss being proportional to the amount of remodeling activity, or bone turnover. A new remodeling cycle begins every ten seconds somewhere in the skeleton of a healthy adult. Each year, between 7 and 10 percent of our entire skeleton is remodeled, serving two purposes: (1) normal growth, and repair and replacement of worn-out and broken bone, and (2) maintenance of normal blood calcium levels.

Osteocytes are branched cells, embedded in the matrix of mineralized bone. They transmit chemical information to surface cells, probably assist in mineral exchange between the matrix and the bloodstream, and generally help keep bone tissue in mint condition.

Bone formation prevails in youth; resorption prevails in the elderly and the inactive, and during certain disease conditions. As we look at bone, it is hard to believe that it is one of the most active tissues of the body, in a constant state of flux, in every stage of construction, in all areas of our skeleton throughout our lifetime.

4

HORMONES

An organism as complex as our body needs a sensitive and exacting method of regulation. *Hormones* are chemical messengers that help perform this vital role. Primarily produced by *endocrine glands* and transported by the bloodstream, they carry messages to distant target tissues, telling them to act in specific ways. Often hormones respond to each other through interdependent feedback. Minute amounts regulate most body processes. In proper balance, they enable systems to work together in harmony for the well-being of the whole body.

Specific glands and hormones play vital roles in the processes of bone formation and loss, metabolism, and calcium utilization.

The **pituitary gland:** This gland lies near the hypothalamus at the base of the brain, and is somewhat controlled by it because its hormones activate pituitary hormones. (They also may influence emotions, eating disorders, and ovulatory and menstrual irregularity.) In turn, pituitary hormones control the activity of other glands. *Thyroid stimulating hormones (TSH)* act on the thyroid gland, *adrenocorticotropic hormones (ACTH)* act on the adrenal glands, and *follicle-stimulating (FSH)* and *luteinizing hormones (LH)* control activities of the sex glands. *Growth hormones (GH)* help regulate growth.

Parathyroid glands: Two glands on each side of the thyroid gland in the neck secrete *parathormone (PTH)*. Along with vitamin D it is the prime regulator of calcium and phosphorus metabolism and demonstrates the finely-tuned feedback system. A dip in blood calcium spurs PTH to take the following actions to raise it back to normal: (1) osteoclasts resorb more bone, releasing calcium and phosphorus into the bloodstream; (2) more calcium is absorbed from food; and (3) kidneys excrete more phosphate, increasing blood calcium.

The **thyroid gland:** This gland lies over the windpipe like a resting butterfly. One hormone, *calcitonin*, acts just the opposite of PTH, inhibiting resorption if blood calcium gets too high. Together their actions maintain blood calcium within a narrow normal range. *Triiodothyronine* (T3) and *Thyroxine* (T4) help control metabolism, stimulate secretion of GH, convert cartilage into bone, assure normal growth and development of the skeleton, and may speed the turnover of bone tissue.

Adrenal glands: Perching like tricorns atop the kidneys, each gland consists of two portions, the *medulla* and the *cortex*. The medulla produces two hormones, adrenaline (epinephrine) and noradrenaline (norepinephrine). At the first sign of distress, they are released into the bloodstream and raise the heart rate and blood pressure. The cortex produces three types of corticosteroids: glucocorticoids (hydrocortisone family), mineralocorticoids (aldosterone), and sex hormones. Most corticosteroids are controlled by a pituitary hormone. Adrenal hormones affect protein, carbohydrate, and fat metabolism, and immune and anti-inflammatory responses.

Gonads: These are the sex glands, the testes in males and the ovaries in females. Hormones direct male and female growth and development, sex characteristics and behavior, skeletal differences, and reproductive function. Testes manufacture male sex hormones called androgens, primarily *testosterone*. Testosterone helps prevent bone loss and may enhance bone building. Ovaries manufacture the potent bone-protecting female sex hormone, *estrogen*, and *progesterone*. Lower levels of all sex hormones are linked to osteoporosis.

Over 30 hormones have been identified since the first was discovered almost a century ago. It is only when hormones are out of balance that we conceive their power to create giants and dwarfs, and cause obesity, diabetes, goiters, and other conditions, among them osteoporosis.

Today most endocrine imbalance is diagnosed and treated before symptoms become severe. Hormones can be extracted from tissue or produced synthetically, offering broad possibilities for application. They are, for example, already used to treat cancer, high blood pressure, and osteoporosis, and to facilitate birth control.

With the recent introduction of recombinant DNA technology, human growth hormone now can be mass-produced, providing a plentiful supply for research purposes. Studies already have revealed the ability of GH to increase lean body mass, break down and reduce fat tissue, and thicken thinning skin. These changes in body composition formerly were considered an inevitable and unavoidable part of the aging process. Now we know they can be reversed by one to two decades with GH treatment. This information opens the door to possible therapeutic uses, especially for older individuals, because atropy of muscle and skin contribute to frailty. For instance, GH may be helpful for certain chronically ill or postoperative patients who can't exercise but need to build muscle. Because GH production declines in postmenopausal women and with age, researchers are exploring connections to osteoporosis that may one day enhance prevention. In Europe, adults who are deficient in GH have shown improved bone density after treatment. Much more research is needed before general use is justified, but the outlook has never been more optimistic.

Studies linking other hormones to osteoporosis also show promise. Keep informed on future breakthroughs; technology is picking up speed, advancing in many areas. As we learn more about hormones, perhaps we can help nature achieve and maintain balance. In the meantime, act on current knowledge to maintain good health.

5

RISK FACTORS: ARE YOU
A LIKELY CANDIDATE?

Risk factors are personal characteristics or circumstances
that render some of us more likely than others to experience a
condition or disease—in this case, osteoporosis. You can
determine if you are a candidate by matching your particular
situation to the following list of risk factors, identified through
years of research. (They will be discussed in greater detail in
later Keys.) If you think you are at risk for osteoporosis, you
should see a doctor and get your bone mass measured.

- Age forty or older
- Female
- Thin, small-boned frame
- Decreased estrogens (from natural, early, or surgically-
  induced menopause)
- Caucasian or Asian
- Use of certain medications, including corticosteroids, thy-
  roid supplements, heparin, loop diuretics (thiazides may
  increase bone mass), anticonvulsants, antacids containing
  aluminum, and tetracycline
- Lack of regular exercise; prolonged immobility
- Calcium deficient diet, including chronic, low-grade cal-
  cium deficiency
- Cigarette smoker
- Family history of osteoporosis
- Heavy alcohol or caffeine intake
- Dietary imbalance (lack of vitamin D; excess protein,
  phosphorus, sodium)
- Related underlying health problems (hormone imbalance,
  gastrointestinal surgery or disease, liver or kidney disease,
  dietary disorders, chronic illnesses)

Are you at risk for osteoporosis? If you are a forty-five-year-old thin white female who smokes, leads a sedentary lifestyle, and whose diet is low in calcium, the process probably has begun already. At age fifty-five, postmenopausal, and given the same circumstances, it probably is present and worsening. By age sixty-five, unless you have made some lifestyle changes and have begun treatment, you probably have obvious signs.

Osteoporosis is characterized by slow bone loss that usually calls attention to itself with the sharp snap of a bone. *Our probability of developing osteoporosis, and therefore our susceptibility to fractures, is related directly to the amount of bone mass, or density, we build and retain.* The peak (maximum) bone mass one can achieve is determined somewhat genetically but, along with bone loss, also is based on a variety of internal and external factors. Thus the strength and density of our bone tissue, and the amount and rate of decline, is subject to change.

Are you on the "suspect" or "pretty sure" end of the risk range? The presence of several risk factors does not mean you have or will develop osteoporosis, or that you will be beseiged by fractures as you get older. Nor does their absence mean you are protected and need not be concerned. It is not known why some people develop osteoporosis, whereas others with similar life conditions do not. Risk factors present a common pattern of predisposition. If you fit the pattern, you are more likely to develop osteoporosis. Exceptions to the rule exist, but you should take risk factors seriously. They are like flashing red lights, urging you to stop, learn—and act.

Some risk factors we can change, some we can possibly change, and some we cannot change. Knowing that osteoporosis is eight times more common in women than in men, we cannot change the fact if we are female. However, we can try to counteract risk factors that are beyond our control. We can stop smoking; limit our intake of alcohol, caffeine, and phosphorus-rich soft drinks; eat a calcium-rich balanced diet; and enjoy regular exercise according to our ability. The incidence of osteoporosis can be cut drastically if we are aware of these truths and practice prevention.

Osteoporosis in itself is a risk factor. Most fractures in older adults result from falls; osteoporosis compounds the peril of falls by increasing the likelihood of fractures when they occur. Falls are the second leading cause of accidental death among women between ages sixty-five and eighty-four and the fourth leading cause of accidental death among men in that age bracket. For people over age eighty-five, falls are the leading cause of accidental death. Most falls are due to a combination of risk factors, among them, environmental hazards, physiological changes, and osteoporosis. Using persons over age seventy-five who lived at home, a Yale University study (Tinnetti 1986) found that persons with four risk factors had a 78 percent chance of falling, whereas those with no risk factors had only an 8 percent chance of falling. Removing or decreasing risk factors for falls is an important step in osteoporosis treatment and will be discussed in other Keys.

Assess your risk for osteoporosis. The more risk factors you have, the greater your risk for developing it. But remember, your genes are not your destiny. One or two risk factors only mean you must work harder to offset their effect. Seeing evidence that you are at risk should motivate you to act. Begin with a visit to your doctor to discuss your risk and perhaps have your bone mass measured.

6

RISK FACTORS YOU
CANNOT CONTROL

The size and structure of our bones greatly depends on our genes. We may be fortunate to have our father's aristocratic nose, but we are just as apt to have the misfortune of our mother's tendency for osteoporosis.

Studies show definite patterns of the incidence of osteoporosis, based on inherited factors. The important roles of race and ethnicity are clearly evident. Our sex, the number of years we live, and the size and density of our bones also affect our likelihood of developing osteoporosis. All are influenced by our parentage—the genes we receive. Even the rate of bone loss may be determined genetically.

According to studies, fair-skinned, petite women of European heritage are at the very highest risk, and black men are at the very lowest risk. The fact that Caucasians and those of Asian ancestry are more likely candidates is linked to their smaller stature. Because women in general are smaller than men, they have about 30 percent less bone mass to begin with. Blacks of both sexes tend to have larger, heavier frames and denser bones, and are less likely to develop osteoporosis. However, lower fracture rates in blacks also have been linked to larger muscle mass from increased physical labor, obesity, differences in calcium utilization, and higher levels of the protective hormone, calcitonin.

Skin pigmentation itself seems to be a factor. Hispanics and those of Mediterranean ancestry are at lower risk than whites. And the lighter the complexion, the more likely are people to succumb. Keep in mind that these are patterns. Each person is unique, and even genetic tendencies are just that—tendencies. However, because osteoporosis is a worldwide health problem, identifying those populations at high risk is of great value in directing care and management.

Your doctor will ask for information to help assess your risk. Is there a history of osteoporosis in your family? If your mother or sister has osteoporosis, you are especially prone. Close relatives who have scoliosis or related types of bone disease also put us at risk. Look through family albums. Is there evidence of bone disease? Were any relatives short? Stooped? Is there a history of fractures? Was Grandma crippled by a fractured hip? Remember, the condition was not apt to be named years ago. Older relatives may not have been diagnosed properly, or may have been unfamiliar with the term osteoporosis. Many of the health problems science is attacking and conquering once were considered the normal course of aging.

We can't dictate our genes as yet, but major advances in genetic structuring may make that possible one day. Until then, we must work to counter negative risk factors that we can control. Take preventive measures to protect yourself and members of your family before spontaneous fractures impose limits. Make certain that osteoporosis does not creep up and steal your independence, mobility, and productivity.

7

AGE-RELATED (SENILE) OSTEOPOROSIS

Osteoporosis is a metabolic disorder in which bone resorption increases while bone formation stays the same or slows. As bones lose minerals, spaces within become larger and bones become fragile and easily broken. Osteoporosis may be primary or secondary to another condition. Two types of primary osteoporosis are recognized: postmenopausal (high turnover) and senile (low turnover). Many factors influence the onset, progress, and severity.

Diagnosis of osteoporosis is complicated; secondary causes must be ruled out. Osteoporosis is considered present when bone mass is less than normal for one's age and sex. However, the threshold between normal and excess bone loss is not well defined. Further, if primary and secondary osteoporosis are both present, a common occurrence, it often is difficult to distinguish between them. Primary osteoporosis is diagnosed only after all other causes of abnormally low bone mass are ruled out.

Senile osteoporosis typically strikes men and women over age sixty-five. Loss of both cortical and trabecular bone primarily results in fractures of the spine and hip, although fractures of the pelvis and other bones also often occur. The vertebral fractures often are of the multiple, wedge type and lead to painless *kyphosis,* or "dowager's hump."

When we are young, bone is built up faster than it is broken down. Although remodeling continues throughout life, between ages thirty and forty, a slow, insidious deterioration, first of trabecular and then cortical bone, begins and progresses unless we act in a disciplined and decisive manner during these "brink" years and beyond.

18

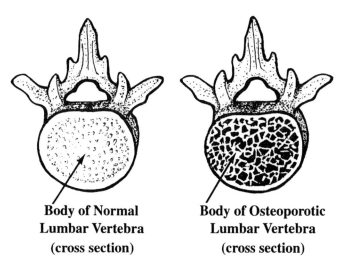

**Body of Normal
Lumbar Vertebra
(cross section)**

**Body of Osteoporotic
Lumbar Vertebra
(cross section)**

Tracing patterns of age-related bone loss, we see that both sexes follow the same general path. Trabecular bone is lost at the rate of approximately 0.5 to 1 percent per year. Cortical bone loss begins almost a decade later and proceeds at the rate of about 0.3 to 0.5 percent a year, increasing slightly over time until it levels off around age sixty-five. Confounded by both postmenopausal and senile osteoporosis, women can lose half of their trabecular bone and over one third of their cortical bone tissue during their lifetime.

Age-related lifestyle and physiological changes are major causal factors, the highway robbers in senile osteoporosis. Flagging physical activity and chronic illnesses are more common in the elderly. The level of the bone-protecting hormone, calcitonin, decreases, whereas parathormone climbs, increasing bone turnover. Vitamin D aids calcium absorption, but as the need for both grows, intake and utilization wane. Older people not only spend less time outdoors, but aging skin is less able to manufacture vitamin D from the sun. Decreased hydrochloric acid in the stomach (10 percent of the elderly have little or none) also hinders calcium absorption. Some people find it hard to digest milk in later life, so they give up calcium-rich milk products to avoid gastric distress. Further, the body's ability to adjust to lower calcium ingestion is impaired by aging. All of these changes serve to advance osteoporosis.

How can you recognize osteoporosis? It is not easy in the beginning stages. Early symptoms of osteoporosis are absent or vague or typical of a multitude of other illnesses. They include weakness, stiffness, a shaky, unsteady gait, and poor appetite. A person may tire more easily and become more irritable. Depression may occur due to chronic pain and increased difficulty performing daily activities. Progressive curvature of the spine, resulting in kyphosis, affects posture, coordination, gait, and balance.

The most common and most debilitating symptom is pain, usually in the mid and lower spine. It may be mild or severe. Sometimes fractures occur and there is no pain at all. Eventually there may be marked changes in the spine, such as nerve damage, severe kyphosis, and loss of height. The size of the chest cavity may be so diminished that breathing is impaired. It is usually back pain or a fracture that finally moves individuals to seek medical attention.

Osteoporosis offers no warning signs yet claims the lives of 40,000 individuals who die from its complications each year, in addition to those who suffer broken bones. The good news is that we don't have to sit back and let it happen. Even in advanced stages, we can take precautions, follow recommended treatments, and reduce or eliminate disability with optimum rehabilitation.

8

MENOPAUSE AND POSTMENOPAUSAL OSTEOPOROSIS

Two types of primary osteoporosis are named in Key 7. We will all have some evidence of senile osteoporosis if we live long enough. Postmenopausal osteoporosis, however, strikes earlier, hits harder, and, of course, attacks only women. Women who understand the bodily changes and hormonal actions involved can make decisions that will remove unnecessary stress, enhance the quality of life, and reduce the risk of bone loss and fracture.

The skeletal and reproductive systems work together to steer both sexual and physical characteristics, beginning just after conception when sex hormones are first secreted. Triggered by a rush of hormones, adolescence begins between ages eleven and fifteen with a season of dramatic physical growth and sexual development called *puberty*. Fusion of long bones begins with the first menstrual period (*menarche*). A glandular chain reaction from the hypothalamus to the pituitary to the ovaries causes estrogen and progesterone production to begin.

Each month, follicle-stimulating and luteinizing hormones prime the ovaries to produce their own hormones and ripen and release eggs. Estrogen levels rise to prepare the uterus for the ovum (egg). Halfway through the cycle, *ovulation* occurs and the egg leaves the ovary to begin the journey through the fallopian tubes. Progesterone joins estrogen to prepare the endometrial bed of the uterus. If an egg is not fertilized, hormone levels fall, menstruation begins, and the *endometrium* is shed. This hormonal action controls reproduction and protects the bones until menopause.

21

Typically, after age forty, hormonal signals become muddled, ovarian function declines, ovulation ceases, estrogen and progesterone levels taper off, and menstrual periods become irregular. Although we associate all of these signs and symptoms with menopause, the body prepares for menopause during the *perimenopausal* years. *Menopause* is literally the final menstrual period. It occurs between ages forty and fifty-five (average, age fifty-one), ushering in the *climacteric*, indeed, the climax of a woman's reproductive years, referred to as the "change of life." The climacteric continues for the next two to ten years, heralding an array of hormonal and metabolic-induced changes.

About 80 percent of all women experience mild to disabling physical and emotional symptoms during the perimenopausal and climacteric years. Without hormone replacement, symptoms may persist up to fifteen years. As some wane or worsen, others may begin. As the vaginal lining becomes thin and dry, intercourse may be painful. The uterus shrinks to half its size, and as muscles stretch, may prolapse into the vagina, causing incontinence (loss of bladder control). Urinary tract infections, constipation, and weight gain are common. Hot flashes, night sweats and chills, and fatigue and mood swings may take place.

Postmenopausal osteoporosis results when bone resorption exceeds formation and there is a disproportionate loss of bone, primarily trabecular tissue. It is caused by a drop in estrogen production, along with other factors associated with menopause, such as impaired vitamin D and calcium utilization. Crumbling trabecular bone (trabecular bone loss may begin in women as early as age thirty) predisposes women to fractures of the vertebrae, fractures of the forearm, and tooth loss due to a shrinking jawbone. Menopause may impose an additional bone loss of 2 to 3 percent every year for up to a decade, after which it slows, until around age seventy when the rate of bone loss returns to premenopausal levels. The incidence of wrist fractures increases until age sixty-five, then levels off; the rate of vertebral fractures, also associated with senile osteoporosis, continues to rise.

Temporary or permanent interruption of ovarian function may occur earlier in life due to systemic disorder or disease, excessive physical activity, stress, disruptive habits (tobacco, alcohol, drugs), and eating disorders (bulimia, anorexia, malnutrition). If damage, disease, or surgical removal of both ovaries causes hormones to quit abruptly, symptoms can be severe. (Estrogen drops to 60 percent of presurgical levels within three hours following surgical removal of the ovaries.) Estrogen replacement usually is started at once. Symptoms are the same whether menopause is natural or otherwise, but early menopause is a potent predictor of osteoporosis and women who experience it, for whatever reason, increase their risk according to the number of added years they are without estrogen protection.

When ovarian function ceases, androgens from the adrenal glands are converted by the body's fat cells into estrone, a form of estrogen, so that our bodies are not totally depleted. The more body fat one has, the more estrone, and the less bone loss, one reason why obese individuals are less subject to osteoporosis.

Although bone-sparing actions are not fully understood, estrogen clearly inhibits bone loss throughout the skeleton. It appears to act with other hormones to promote calcium absorption, aid calcium and protein metabolism, prompt calcitonin production, and stimulate the liver to produce proteins that bind adrenal hormones, preventing their bone-dissolving effects. On a local level, bone cells contain estrogen receptors, where estrogen may directly decrease the activation of new bone-remodeling units. Because all estrogen-deficient women do not develop postmenopausal osteoporosis, yet unknown factors must be involved, a subject of further research. Progesterone probably prevents adrenal hormones from attaching to bone cell receptors and thus inhibits their bone resorbing ability.

9

SECONDARY CAUSES OF OSTEOPOROSIS

In up to 20 percent of cases in women and 40 percent of cases in men, osteoporosis occurs secondary to another medical problem. This condition could be the sole cause, or could heighten osteoporotic changes already present. For example, long-term steroid treatment of arthritis can cause osteoporosis in healthy bone. On the other hand, gastric bypass or stapling surgery for severe obesity will compound postmenopausal bone loss. Conditions, diseases, and hormonal disturbances that can cause or intensify osteoporosis follow. If any are present in your life and you are at risk or have signs of osteoporosis, discuss your concerns with your doctor. If you are not at risk, but have low bone mass, one of these conditions may be the cause. Careful diagnosis is critical, especially when several disease processes are present.

Imbalance of the very hormones that promote proper bone growth and development can lead to osteoporosis. This includes conditions that inhibit ovarian function, such as stress, excessive exercise, eating disorders, and use of tobacco, alcohol, or certain drugs. Increased (hyperfunction) or decreased (hypofunction) activity of glands commonly is caused by tumors, inflammation, or tissue damage due to surgery or trauma. Thyroid hormones labor to prevent excessive breakdown of bone, but an overactive thyroid gland (hyperthyroidism, thyrotoxicosis, Graves' disease) or treatment for underactivity with thyroid medication, can disturb the balance of calcium and phosphorus and cause osteoporosis. In hyperparathyroidism, excessive amounts of parathormone cue osteoclasts to dig more tunnels than osteoblasts can fill, speeding bone resorption. Bones rapidly become thin and weak, and break with the slightest stress.

Long-term uncontrolled diabetes, a disease marked by a deficiency of the insulin hormone, may lead to osteoporosis. Insulin-dependent diabetics have 10 percent less bone mass than comparable nondiabetics due to increased resorption, especially during the first few years after diagnosis. Decreased bone formation and impaired kidney function also may be contributing factors.

Cushing's syndrome or disease results from overproduction of glucocorticoids by the adrenal glands, either because of adrenal dysfunction, or secondary to pituitary hyperfunction. Osteoporosis is most prominent in spinal and pelvic bones. This is a potentially fatal disease that demands prompt treatment. Hypogonadism is associated with vertebral fractures. In most cases of hormonal imbalance, diagnosis is easy to confirm and treatment can be successfully achieved.

Except for osteoarthritis, which tends to decrease the risk of osteoporosis if proper exercise is continued, the many types of arthritis often are accompanied by osteoporosis. Several reasons are probable. Stiff, painful, or inflamed joints may limit weight-bearing activity, and along with muscle wasting from disuse, predispose one to osteoporosis, especially in long bones. Further, corticosteroids and antacids that often are prescribed interfere with calcium absorption and use; steroids promote bone loss. (Rheumatoid arthritis tops the risk list. Those with rheumatoid arthritis average 10 percent less calcium in their bones than similar non-arthritic individuals.)

Any lung condition that decreases the body's oxygen and nutrient supply, or causes sufficient shortness of breath to limit activity, puts bones in jeopardy. Patients with emphysema (chronic obstructive pulmonary disease) often develop osteoporosis. Cigarette smokers double their risk. It begins earlier, progresses faster, and is more severe. Tobacco use lowers estrogen production and calcium absorption. Women who smoke typically begin menopause five years earlier, snuffing out five years of estrogen protection. The fact that smokers tend to be underweight boosts the risk a step higher. Cigarette smoking is the single most important preventable cause of death. Seek help if necessary, but stop smoking! Discourage young people from developing the habit. Major benefits are realized no matter what age one quits.

Faulty absorption of nutrients from the digestive tract can be due to gastric bypass or stapling, partial removal of the stomach or small intestine, malabsorption, or chronic intestinal diseases. Eating disorders that may cause nutritional and hormonal deficiencies include malnutrition and *anorexia nervosa* (excessive dieting) or *bulimia nervosa* (binge eating and purging). A diseased pancreas may not supply digestive enzymes necessary for the metabolism of calcium and vitamin D. A malfunctioning liver may fail to convert vitamin D to the usable form. Kidney problems may prevent proper calcium excretion and reabsorption. Nutritional disorders can precipitate bone loss. Correcting the condition, adjusting nutrients, or both, usually will alleviate the hazard.

Osteoporosis can be caused both by too little (Key 35) or too much exercise. Although overexercise is uncommon in men, those who combine vigorous training, for example, marathon runners, with an inadequate diet, can lower their testosterone level to the point where bone loss occurs. Women who participate in activities that require trim bodies—runners, ballet dancers, models, jockeys—may lose body fat, stop menstruating, and experience rapid calcium depletion and bone loss. A return to an adequate diet and reasonable level of exercise will reverse the process. (In a University of British Columbia, Vancouver study, women who missed just one menstrual period over 12 months lost 4 percent of bone density a year.) A study of girls, aged thirteen to twenty years, concluded that thin, white, non-menstruating young females engaged in strenuous physical activity over a long period are especially prone to lower bone mineral density (Dhuper, 1990). Precious bone, once lost, may never be replaced.

10

DRUGS THAT CAN CAUSE OSTEOPOROSIS

Some medications that are prescribed for other medical problems, as well as certain over-the-counter (OTC) drugs, alcohol, and caffeine, can lead to osteoporosis if they are used over a period of months or years. Calcium needs will increase and supplements may be prescribed, along with other medications, to offset the effects of these drugs.

Adrenal steroids: These medications, both natural and synthetic, are major offenders. They act by attaching to receptors on bone, promoting bone resorption. Anti-inflammatory properties and the ability to diminish immune responses make them valuable drugs to treat asthma, arthritis, skin diseases, allergic reactions, cancer, and organ transplants. Unfortunately, side effects pose a great threat to bone. Corticosteroids decrease calcium absorption and bone formation and increase calcium excretion and bone loss. (Inhaled, or injected locally to treat an acute condition, they are not likely to cause a problem.) Precautions to minimize the danger of steroid-induced osteoporosis include use of the lowest dose of short-acting steroids for the shortest period of time needed to treat the primary disease, adequate calcium and vitamin D intake, and the use of bone-sparing agents such as estrogens, thiazides, bisphosphonates, and calcitonin.

Alcohol: Interfering with absorption and metabolism of calcium, alcohol decreases production of estrogen and testosterone, and reduces bone formation by direct action on osteoblasts. Alcoholics are also more prone to fractures due to falls, often lack proper nutrition, and may suffer severe bone loss. Omit alcohol altogether (like sugar, it is empty calories), or limit your intake to one or two drinks a day.

27

Caffeine: This stimulant increases calcium excretion in amounts proportional to the amount of caffeine consumed. In one study, the 450 mg of caffeine found in 3 daily cups of coffee resulted in a 28 mg calcium loss. (A 40 mg daily deficit of calcium can produce a 1 to 1.5 percent yearly loss in skeletal mass in postmenopausal women.) Tea, soft drinks, cocoa, and chocolate also contain caffeine. Caffeine is a stimulant drug and users can develop a dependence. (Instant coffee has less caffeine than regular.) It is a good idea to consume no more than one or two caffeinated drinks a day. Taper off over several days. Even one-cup-a-day coffee drinkers may experience side effects with sudden withdrawal: nausea, headaches, anxiety, irritability, drowsiness, depression, and irregular heartbeats.

Aluminum-containing antacids, used to neutralize stomach acid in cases of ulcers and heartburn, can lessen calcium absorption, speed its excretion, and lead to bone demineralization. Six months or more of therapy with the blood thinner, heparin, can lead to osteoporosis. **Phenytoin** (Dilantin), used for seizure control, hampers the liver's ability to metabolize vitamin D, so less calcium is absorbed. Certain diuretics, such as **furosemide,** flush away calcium along with the unwanted fluid that collects in tissues. **Thyroid supplements**, given when thyroid hormones are lacking, can stimulate bone resorption and prompt bone loss. **Tetracycline**, an antibiotic, is absorbed and stored in bone tissue where it interferes with bone growth and metabolism.

These and other medications can interfere with calcium utilization and decrease bone mass. Review your medication use periodically with your doctor. Dosages may require adjustment. Better drugs may become available that are equally effective and are not as harmful to bones or other tissue. Your needs change. Insist on proper monitoring for adverse effects.

The proliferation of drugs and of multiple drug use makes correct use of drugs especially critical. To prevent conflicting treatment, keep a record of all medicine you take, including vitamins, drops, ointments and creams (see sample at the end of this Key). Inform your doctors of any allergic reactions you have had and of all medications you are taking, both prescription and OTC.

These tips will help you manage your medicine and control your health:

- Know the name, purpose, desired effects, and possible side effects of your medicine and when, how, and how long you are to take it.
- Take all drugs exactly as prescribed. Some interact with certain foods; others irritate the stomach unless taken with meals. Some cannot be crushed.
- Take the smallest dose necessary for a therapeutic effect. Sometimes you can treat your symptoms in a more healthy way. For example, constipation often can be relieved with dietary fiber and exercise instead of a laxative.
- Never stop taking prescribed medicine on your own, even if you feel better.
- Never share drugs with others.
- Discard old and unused drugs by flushing them down the toilet.
- Mixing drugs with alcohol can be deadly; caffeine and smoking alter the body's reaction to some drugs. Check if drugs you take are affected.
- Rely on your pharmacist to keep a drug profile, check OTC drugs for possible interaction with your prescription drugs, and provide information and advice.
- Advise your doctor of any unexpected drug reaction.

It is estimated that over half of the 1.6 billion prescriptions written each year are misused, probably because of a lack of knowledge regarding proper management. All drugs have both good and bad aspects; none are totally safe. But they are necessary and often lifesaving. Use sound judgment and never introduce a drug into your body unless you know what you are doing and why.

Medicine Record for Sarah Williams

Name of drug (Generic/Brand)	Ordered by	Date Started	Reason	Form	Daily Dose	Time of day	Side effects to watch for	Special Considerations
Digoxin	Dr. Lee	2-6-90	strengthen and slow heartbeat	tablet	0.125 mg	10 A.M	slow pulse	Inform doctor if pulse is below 60 beats per minute

11

MEN AND OSTEOPOROSIS

Greater bone mass and slower bone loss with age are important reasons why men are less likely than women to develop osteoporosis, at least not until they are much older. The advantage of larger bones begins in childhood, when boys enjoy more leisurely time to stretch and grow. Although they begin puberty later, typically boys already are taller than girls, grow faster and bigger, and continue growing longer, into their twenties.

While adolescent girls deal with increased levels of estrogen and progesterone, boys struggle with their own sex hormones. Just as the pituitary gland sends hormones to spur the ovaries to action, its luteinizing hormones also stimulate the testes to produce sperm, male hormones, and small quantities of estrogens. Testosterone production is further regulated by the hypothalamus. Whereas girls develop fat tissue and figures, adolescent boys develop dense bones, and strong muscles and physiques (in part due to more strenuous physical labor).

Male sex hormones, called androgens, flow at a fairly steady rate. They are responsible for male reproductive function and physical and behavioral characteristics, such as a deep voice, broad shoulders, and aggressiveness. The endocrine system releases the proper type and amount of hormones at just the right time to assure normal development. (Androgens from the adrenal glands have little impact in males.) Testosterone, the primary male hormone, plays a major role in developing and maintaining large muscles and dense bones. A male humerus (upper armbone), for example, is one-third more dense than that of a female.

Testosterone probably enhances bone building and plays a role similar to estrogen in preventing bone loss. Low testosterone levels and low bone mineral density are conditions found in alcoholism and in hypogonadism in men; both also are associated with osteoporosis.

The following factors also work to the male advantage, at least until around age sixty-five:

- Slower rate of bone loss
- Decreased loss of lateral bracing trabeculae
- Higher levels of calcitonin
- Higher consumption of calcium
- More weight-bearing exercise
- No rapid hormonal decline comparable to menopause

Although the supply of testosterone slows over time, the overall decline is not great enough to cause large amounts of bone loss. It is only around age sixty or sixty-five that men really begin to succumb to primary osteoporosis. Studies show that of the 20 to 30 percent of vertebral bone mass that men lose during their lifetime, more than half is lost after age sixty. (On the other hand, of the 45 to 50 percent of vertebral bone mass that women lose during their lifetime, most is lost between ages forty-five and sixty.) One out of every five persons who has osteoporosis is male. By extreme old age, one out of six men will sustain a hip fracture.

Because osteoporosis is, to a great extent, a woman's health problem, most research has been done among women. Generally, however, findings regarding diet, exercise, environment, and other factors that affect the risks of osteoporosis in women show similiar risks for men.

12

YOUTH AND OSTEOPOROSIS

Except in rare instances, osteoporosis is virtually unheard of in youth. *Juvenile osteoporosis* in prepubescent children causes heel, ankle, and lower back pain and severe bone loss for a period of two to four years. The cause is unknown and symptoms usually disappear spontaneously followed by resumption of bone growth. Another form of primary osteoporosis that occurs in young adults causes mainly vertebral fractures and is called *idiopathic osteoporosis. Osteogenesis imperfecta*, sometimes called brittle bone disease, is a hereditary disorder that primarily affects bone, causing fractures to occur in infancy and resulting in varying degrees of deformity. Babies and children who are bedridden for long periods due to fractures often develop osteoporosis due to immobility.These conditions are rare. If osteoporosis occurs in youth, it is usually because of other problems, such as hormonal or nutritional imbalance, prolonged immobilization, or drugs.

Although we associate osteoporosis with old age, we will triumph over osteoporosis only if we redirect attention to the beginning years of life. Youth offers the opportunity to assess hereditary factors and establish healthy habits that will deter osteoporosis. Our important role as mature adults is to educate and enable youth, to start them on the right road—the road to peak bone mass.

To encourage organized physical activity may seem redundant when youngsters seem to never sit still. Yet, as we get older, a habit of regular physical exercise established in childhood serves our greatest interests. As communities struggle with rising school budgets, the temptation is to cut corners on gyms and playing fields. Make sure that the youth in your community have access to a variety of physical activities and encourage active play and participation in organized sports. Lifelong sports like tennis and cycling are especially useful.

A balanced diet that includes adequate calcium and protein is critical, especially during the rapid growth periods. Most children have fairly adequate diets until they reach those trying teen years when risk factors increase, along with pressures from peers and parents, school and society—and from within. Smoking, drinking alcohol, overconsumption of soft drinks and fast foods, and frequent dieting pose particular problems in adolesence and should be discouraged.

Two conditions are especially dangerous: eating disorders and teen pregnancy. Eating disorders are exacerbated by society's obsession with "thin," although studies suggest hypothalmic, genetic, psychiatric, and other influences. An estimated 10 percent of females, almost exclusively adolescent girls and young women, suffer from anorexia nervosa, self-induced starvation, and bulimia nervosa, characterized by binge eating and purging by vomiting and/or excessive use of laxatives and diuretics. They are often intelligent overachievers from upper middle-class families who see themselves as fat even when they actually are suffering life-threatening emaciation; 2 percent die of starvation or complications. Lifestyles that demand low weight pose a special threat.

Changes occur in all systems as the body tries to protect itself. Extreme weight loss can disrupt ovarian activity, causing skipped menstrual periods or none at all (*amenorrhea*). Bone loss follows. A study (Mazess et al. 1990) of 11 female patients with anorexia found a 22 to 27 percent reduction of spinal bone mineral density. Although some bone tissue can be regained if the condition is treated successfully and menstruation returns to normal, recovery probably is not complete. Consistently attempt to build self-esteem and persuade victims to get professional help.

34

Teenage pregnancy places both the mother's bones, which are still growing and developing, as well as the baby's bones in jeopardy. Lacking adequate calcium (1,600 mg daily), pregnant and lactating adolescents lose bone minerals, fail to develop peak bone mass, and are more likely to develop osteoporosis at an earlier age.

Teens and their parents should know the special risks that accompany the "growing years." Adolescents and young women who have stopped menstruating for whatever reason should seek medical help to keep their bones healthy. Peak bone mass can be achieved only if calcium intake is adequate. Calcium supplements may be necessary for those who cannot or will not drink milk.

Typically, when we are young we see ourselves as unbreakable and eternal. Disease and disability are strangers, except as they apply to others. We cannot envision being in a wheelchair or being bedridden by a hip fracture. We turn deaf ears to advice from our elders about the tenuousness of life.

If healthy habits that prevent bone loss are formed during childhood, and continued throughout life, osteoporosis will be as rare at age eighty as it is at age eight.

13

MEDICAL SPECIALISTS AND MEDICAL TESTS

Ironically, early attention to osteoporosis is both crucial and frequently unattended to because there simply are no symptoms. Waiting until the first sign of osteoporosis occurs, typically a broken bone, allows the disease to progress to a degree that places bones in severe jeopardy. Fortunately, early detection is becoming more prevalent as the public gains knowledge of osteoporosis.

In a society of health specialties and subspecialties, to whom do you address your concerns? Begin with your primary physician, usually a family practitioner or internist. A steward of your health, ideally this person knows your medical history, your lifestyle as it relates to your health, and your special needs. He or she will assess your risk factors, look for changes in height and posture (measure yourself every six months to note any height loss), recommend preventive measures, order tests, and prescribe treatment when indicated. Together you will make plans and decisions that will assure your optimum health.

Your primary physician also acts as gatekeeper, consulting with other physicians, making referrals to specialists, and generally coordinating your care. Specialists who are knowledgeable about osteoporosis include the following:

Gynecologist: A doctor trained to treat conditions that affect the female reproductive system. Women in their forties, as menopause approaches, should consult a gynecologist about issues associated with estrogen deficiency.

Endocrinologist: A specialist in disorders of the endocrine system. An endocrinologist is well suited to evaluate the effect of hormones on bone metabolism and diagnose and treat metabolic conditions, such as osteoporosis, especially if there is a question regarding their cause.

Rheumatologist: This medical specialist is concerned with the development, preservation, and restoration of form and function of the musculoskeletal system, especially as it relates to pain and other symptoms of disease, such as inflammation, degeneration, or metabolic disturbances.

Orthopedist: A specialist in the medical treatment of the skeletal system, its joints, muscles, and associated structures.

Orthopedic surgeon: A specialist who treats the surgical aspects of the musculoskeletal system.

Physiatrist: A specialist in physical medicine, trained in rehabilitation.

Tests that measure bone density (Key 14), the following tests, and others may be used to detect osteoporosis, fractures, and fracture potential, assess the progress of treatment, and rule out other conditions with similar symptoms.

X ray: This is usually the first diagnostic tool used because osteoporosis is often first diagnosed when a conventional X ray, taken for other purposes, reveals old fractures. Although wedging and other changes in bone shape are clear, from 25 to 40 percent of the bone mass must be gone before the loss can be detected by X ray. X rays are more valuable in the diagnosis of fracture than of osteoporosis. (The cost of an X ray of an extremity is $35 to $80; of a spine, $50 to $150.)

Neutron activation: This is a more complex X ray method that measures the total amount of calcium in the body. Repeated at intervals, it is a good indicator of bone loss or gain. Unfortunately, the test is expensive, available only at large medical centers, and is used mainly for research.

Bone scan: This test identifies fractures by marking unusual bone activity and most often is used to rule out other kinds of bone disease. A small amount of a radioactive material injected into a vein collects in bone tissue. A special camera scans the body and records patterns of radioactivity in the form of images. Areas of increased radioactivity, or "hot spots," indicate new bone formations occurring at the site of recent compression fractures. The tiny amount of radionuclide you receive is eliminated from your body in one to two days and poses no danger.

Bone biopsy: This test involves removal of a bone sample containing both cortical and trabecular tissue for microscopic examination. It is an expensive and invasive procedure, causes discomfort, and is not a reliable means to diagnose osteoporosis. It can be useful in difficult cases and may be used to rule out other bone diseases, such as osteomalacia.

Endometrial biopsy: This test is done periodically when estrogen therapy without progesterone is used to treat osteoporosis. A sampling of the endometrial lining is obtained during a pelvic examination in your doctor's office. Mild cramping during the procedure and slight uterine bleeding for several days afterwards may occur.

Biochemical markers of bone turnover revealed in blood and urine tests help identify other health problems that accompany, cause, or mimic osteoporosis; provide information about bone metabolism and remodeling; and can be of help in monitoring the body's response to treatment. The following tests and others may be ordered:

Blood test: Tests may include analysis for calcium, phosphorus, cell counts, alkaline phosphatase, protein electrophoresis, thyroid and parathyroid hormones, and vitamin D levels. These tests are within normal limits in osteoporosis, however, they are of value to detect secondary causes and underlying conditions, such as a vitamin D deficiency, thyroid or parathyroid hyperactivity, kidney or liver disease, and other bone disorders, such as Paget's disease, osteomalacia, or cancer.

Urine test: A test done primarily to determine protein, calcium, and hydroxyproline levels. By measuring hydroxyproline, an amino acid formed during bone resorption, it is possible to determine the amount of calcium being absorbed by the body. A 24-hour urine collection may be required.

14

BONE MASS MEASUREMENT: DENSITOMETRY

No single test determines just *when* our bones bow to osteoporosis, but science has provided a technology to detect its presence in its earliest stages. Densitometry makes it possible to measure both trabecular and cortical bone, identify low bone mineral density (BMD), predict future fracture risk, and monitor changes in bone mass to determine the success of treatment. Four basic techniques have been developed: single photon absorptiometry (SPA), dual photon absorptiometry (DPA), dual energy X ray absorptiometry (DXA), and quantitative computed tomography (QCT).

Testing is becoming more readily available, but not everyone has easy access. However, your doctor can make arrangements without great difficulty. It is not necessary to know each method. Changing technology will likely bring newer and better ones. Simply know what tests are available, something about the techniques involved, when they are appropriate, and how to access them. Some techniques are used mainly for research. All are safe; the radiation dose is low (with the exception of QCT). They are convenient; no preparation is necessary. The procedures are noninvasive; no needles, tubes, or injections are used. And the procedures are comfortable—unless a brief period on an examination table causes distress. Some people fall asleep.

Single Photon Absorptiometry (SPA)

This simple procedure takes about 20 minutes and typically measures the radius in the forearm, although other bones, such as a heel or finger, may be used. A small device scans the area, registering on a computer printout the amount of bone mineral in its path. Because radiation exposure is minute, this technique can be repeated safely over time to monitor the rate of bone loss or to assess the efficacy of treatment.

Because the forearm contains large amounts of cortical bone, and fracture sites in the spine and hip are mainly trabecular bone, some researchers question the ability of SPA to predict the risk of fracture in these areas. However, most researchers agree that these studies do provide a valid prediction of bone mass throughout the body. SPA was the first test developed, is less precise than newer tests, and now is used mainly for research purposes.

Dual Photon Absorptiometry (DPA)

DPA is similar to SPA, but is more sophisticated. This technique can be used to scan thicker body parts, such as the spine and the hip. It also can scan the entire skeleton to measure total body bone mineral. As the individual lies on a table, a scanner passes over the target area. Radioactive material emits photons at two different energies to measure actual bone mass and prints out the BMD for evaluation. In addition to a quantitative analysis, the computer will produce an image of the spine, indicating by color the mineral levels of the vertebrae. DPA takes about 30 minutes and is accurate, precise, and accessible to most people. It can be repeated safely because radiation dose is low, one-tenth that of a routine chest X ray.

Dual Energy X ray Absorptiometry (DXA)

DXA is a more advanced DPA technique that uses an X ray tube instead of radioactive material as a measuring source. DXA enables more precise BMD measurement; produces clearer, better quality images; reduces scanning time to less than ten minutes; and uses a low dose of radiation. Newer applications, such as lateral spine scanning, have been developed. DXA represents a major advance in the field of densitometry and undoubtedly will be the method of choice as it becomes more widely available.

Quantitative Computed Tomography (QCT)

CT scanners, operated in a quantitative rather than an imaging mode, enable separate analysis of trabecular and cortical bone. While lying on a movable table that passes through the "hole" of a large doughnut-shaped machine, detailed cross sections of body parts are obtained by transmission of very thin X ray beams. The cross sections are measured and recorded by a computer. Specific areas then can be analyzed to determine density. QCT is used primarily to measure the spine. QCT scans are expensive, and although the radiation dose is not excessive, it is approximately 50 times greater than DXA, an important consideration if repeated measurements are planned.

The frequency of testing depends on the reason for follow-up. For example, if a bone measurement done when a woman is going through menopause is within a normal range, retesting may be done in two or three years. If the initial test indicates that she is one who is prone to rapid bone loss, six months is more reasonable. The SPA, DPA, and DXA can be repeated safely. Always weigh benefits against risks. In the case of osteoporosis, potential benefits make the decision for testing a wise one.

Other bone measurement techniques either are not widely applicable or still are being developed. None are reimbursable. Compton scattering, a technique that also uses high-energy photons from a radioactive source, currently is being tested in research centers. Ultrasound uses sound waves and their echos to measure stages of bone density much like the sonar system on ships. Because sound waves move more quickly through denser bone, it is also possible to detect fracture. Magnetic resonance imaging (MRI) uses radio waves and magnetic fields to do sophisticated analysis. These and other methods possibly will find wider use.

15

BONE MASS MEASUREMENT: TESTING OR SCREENING

Bone density is the best predictor of whether there is a fracture in your future: the lower your bone mass, the higher your risk. Densitometry tests are used to identify low bone mass, assess bone strength, and predict a future fracture with a moderate degree of accuracy. Thus steps can be taken to prevent fractures from occurring.

Now that screening capabilities are available, that is, the ability to test large segments of the population, is densitometry a viable weapon in the war on osteoporosis? Because osteoporosis is a serious public health problem, is it reasonable to expect at least selective screening, for example, testing white and Asian women who are at or near menopause?

Controversy surrounds this issue. Although densitometry is used to confirm osteoporosis, it is not considered a true diagnostic test, but rather a determinant of risk factor; the fracture itself defines the disease. A measurement of low bone mass is useful to predict the likelihood of fracture much as a measurement of high blood pressure is a risk factor, useful to predict the likelihood of a stroke.

The time to measure bone mineral content (BMC) is when you are considering intervention. Knowledge of the severity of bone loss helps doctors determine appropriate treatment. However, if someone cannot or will not accept treatment, or does not comply with treatment or the necessary follow-up, the role of densitometry is unclear. For some, conscientious attention to diet and safety measures may be of greater value. Although doctors are most likely to recommend hormone replacement for menopausal women unless contraindicated, they are not likely to recommend BMC measurement unless their patient is undecided about taking hormones. On the other hand, if an anorexic woman can see what her eating habits are doing to her bones, is she more apt to accept treatment? Studies show that people who are shown evidence of low bone mass and educated about the repercussions are more easily persuaded to accept and comply with treatment. Too often doctors, too, fail to act until there is evidence that something is wrong.

Cost is another stumbling block to widespread testing. Charges depend on the method used, and the area of the country. SPA may cost from $50 to $75; QCT, $100 to $250. The average cost nationally for a single test is about $100 to $125. Charges may be reduced as part of screening for other conditions. Unfortunately, the high standard of health care we have come to expect is inaccessible to many people who do not have the means to pay.

Reimbursement varies. Most private insurance carriers cover bone density studies, following individual guidelines as to how much coverage is extended and under what circumstances. Presently, Medicare covers only SPA and QCT studies, but this may soon change. The National Osteoporosis Foundation (NOF) and the American Osteoporosis Alliance have attracted congressional attention with lobbying efforts and also have petitioned the Health Care Financing Administration to review their policies on coverage. Call or write to your representatives to encourage their support of legislation for osteoporosis research and funding.

The Scientific Advisory Board of the National Osteoporosis Foundation recommends bone mass measurements for the following:

- To help make decisions about hormone replacement therapy in estrogen-deficient women. Although other factors must be considered, low bone mass would direct what treatment is advisable and provide motivation to follow it.
- To diagnose osteoporosis in persons who have abnormalities of the spine and X ray evidence of bone loss, to aid

decision making regarding further diagnostic evaluation and therapy.

- To diagnose low bone mass in persons who are receiving long-term glucocorticoid therapy, in order to initiate proper treatment or adjust therapy.
- To diagnose low bone mass in persons with primary asymptomatic hyperparathyroidism, to identify those who are at risk of severe skeletal disease and may be candidates for surgical intervention.

Unfortunately, there is no way to measure money that might be saved if low bone mass were noted on a screening test and proper intervention prevented a fracture from occurring, much less to measure the pain and suffering and the deaths that would be averted. A doctor will use a stress test to see if your heart is up to the task before you begin aerobics to prevent a heart attack, but is unlikely to order a bone mass measurement to see if your bones are up to a program of weight-lifting to prevent osteoporosis. Treatment for a fractured hip is about $15,000, with permanent nursing home placement a reality in many cases, at a yearly cost of about $35,000. Screening programs, at least among high risk populations, would encourage therapeutic intervention that would help reduce the cost, monetary and otherwise, of disease and death that results from undetected osteoporosis.

Diagnosis and treatment of osteoporosis is not based on bone measurement alone, but on a comprehensive health evaluation. Screening is neither appropriate nor necessary in many instances, but as treatment options grow, and if the value of densitometry in fracture prevention is confirmed by further studies, guidelines probably will be redefined. Whereas prevention of osteoporosis should be universal, for the majority of us who have passed the fifth decade of our life with minimal knowledge and less than adequate attention to the health of our bones, prevention of fractures is now a major goal. Densitometry may open a window of hope, enabling us to reach our goal.

16

FRACTURES

A *fracture* is a crack or break in a bone. Eighty percent of the 1.3 million fractures that occur each year are related to reduced bone mass, the hallmark of osteoporosis. Bones typically break when they are stressed by a force greater than they can withstand. Osteoporotic bones may snap like dry twigs with normal stress. Osteoporotic fractures usually occur in the femur, the vertebrae, and the wrist. In one in five cases, a broken bone is the cause rather than the result of a fall.

It is not always easy to tell if a bone is broken. Evaluate all pain, especially if it follows activity. Look for these signs and symptoms of fracture:
- A fall, bump, blow, or other trauma, or sudden pain or discomfort during a bending or twisting movement
- Pain that is intensified by movement or weight-bearing
- Swelling or bruising over a bone
- Deformity of the affected limb
- Loss of function in the area of the injury
- Bone poking through the skin
- The sound of a bone cracking

All fractures require immediate first aid and medical follow-up. In most cases an X ray confirms the diagnosis, but not always. Hairline fractures may barely be visible. The *computed tomography* (CT) scan is used to detect fractures of complex areas like the hip, pelvis, and spine.

Treatment is by *closed* (traction) or *open* (surgical) *reduction,* depending primarily on the nature of the fracture. In closed reduction, the doctor manipulates bone parts and "reduces," or "sets" them back into correct position. Realigned bone is immobilized with a bandage, splint, or cast. Sometimes small incisions are made and bones are fixed in place with pins attached to an external frame. In open reduction, an incision is made and bones are set into proper position and fixed in place with hardware: pins, wires, plates, screws, nails, or rods. The purpose of *traction* is to relieve muscle spasm, move bone ends into normal alignment, and immobilize them. Immobilization reduces pain, prevents further damage, and holds broken pieces of bone in close contact while healing takes place.

After treatment and immobilization of a fracture, medical personnel teach, direct, and assist with follow-up care. Those who sustain a fracture and all who are involved in their care should understand and be able to manage the following:

- Care of casts and other immobilizing devices
- Prevention of skin breakdown, swelling, and infection
- Proper use of prescribed and OTC medication for pain relief and healing
- Restriction of activities and movement
- Modification of activities of daily living, including personal hygiene
- Safe use of assistive devices that aid walking and enable progressive levels of activity
- Program of progressive exercise and activity prescribed by a doctor and learned in therapy

The moment a bone is broken, our body begins to repair the damage. Blood clots form. White cells remove dead tissue and debris. When the cleanup is completed, bone-forming osteoblasts multiply and produce and deposit protein matrix and other materials, fashioning a collar of fresh bone (*callus*) that extends above and below the fracture line. Osteoclasts and osteoblasts remodel the callus to its normal shape as bone gradually heals together. As new cells and mineral crystals are deposited in the matrix, the callus hardens, or *ossifies*, into true bone, uniting the parts and closing the gap.

Healing time depends primarily on these factors:

- Type of bone. Each bone has its own healing time. Immobilization needed for union is *approximately* as follows:

fractures of the wrist, six to ten weeks; fractures of the vertebrae, two to three months; and fractures of the femur, three to six months or more. A new technique that applies tiny electric currents to bones has proven successful in speeding the healing process in some cases.

- Extent of injury. An inadequate blood supply, infection, and the movement of bone fragments disrupts normal callus formation. Shattered bones require extensive surgery and may take a year or more to heal. In very rare cases, bones may never heal together properly.
- Age and general health. Chronic conditions may affect the rate of healing and success of rehabilitation. For example, someone with diabetes may not heal as rapidly; one who has disabling arthritis may need a modified rehabilitation program.

Bone scans and *magnetic resonance imaging (MRI)* scans can detect complications, such as nonunion, infection, and damage to the blood and nerve supply. Other complications associated with fracture include disuse atrophy, pneumonia, and blood clot formation.

The goals of treatment after a fracture are to relieve pain, prevent complications, and return the individual to the level of activity enjoyed prior to fracture.

17

FRACTURES OF THE HIP AND WRIST

Each year, more than 300,000 Americans sustain osteoporotic fractures of the hip; 80 percent are women. Of those who do:

- 20 percent will not walk during the first year
- 50 percent will never again walk independently
- 20 percent will require placement in a long-term facility
- 20 percent will die from complications within one year
- Nearly half of frail elderly will die within one year from complications of the fracture or immobility.

Fracture of the Hip

Hip fractures associated with osteoporosis are in the upper part of the femur: the neck and near the trochanteric processes. The head of the femur fits snugly into the cup-shaped socket, or acetabulum, of the pelvic bone. Fracture of the neck requires immediate attention because the blood supply is easily impaired and tissue death (necrosis) may occur. The trochanteric area where the neck joins the shaft of the bone is blessed with a rich blood supply that aids healing and lessens the danger.

Signs and symptoms of a fracture include pain in the hip, thigh, or groin that worsens with movement, reluctance to move or bear weight, and a leg drawn toward the body, rotated outward, and shortened. Any shortening of the affected leg must be evaluated. Pain may be minimal. Individuals have waited several days before seeking treatment and even walked with a fractured hip. Do not move or try to straighten an injured leg or hip that is oddly positioned. *If there is any question of a broken bone, seek medical help.*

48

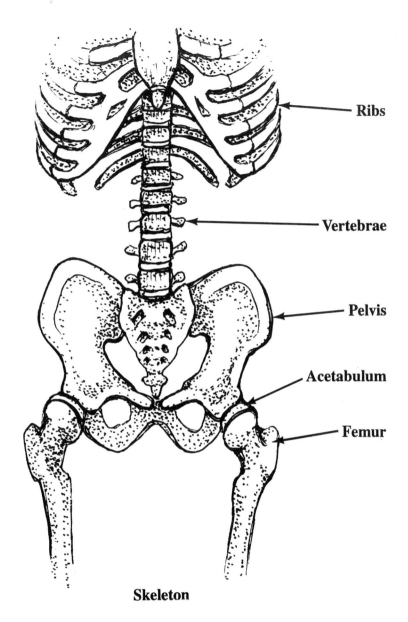

Ribs

Vertebrae

Pelvis

Acetabulum

Femur

Skeleton

Dangerous complications may develop if proper treatment is not provided, or if treatment is delayed.

A doctor will assess the condition, X-ray the injured area, and treat any medical problems. In most cases, surgical repair, which promotes early mobility, is the treatment of choice.

49

The head of the femur may be replaced by an artificial (prosthetic) device. Bed exercises begin almost immediately. Patients are encouraged to do things for themselves at the earliest possible moment to reduce feelings of dependency and motivate progress toward independence. The doctor will order therapy to start as soon as possible, dependent on individual circumstances.

Hip fractures are especially devastating to elderly persons. The fall that causes the fracture is often painful and frightening in itself. In very old individuals, the shock produced by the fracture may be sufficient to cause death within a few days. Major surgery is riskier due to a more frail health status. An already diminished blood or nerve supply slows the healing process. Prolonged bedrest can lead to a variety of complications: pneumonia, bed sores, bladder infection, joint stiffness, bone and muscle atrophy, blood clot formation, and mental confusion. The good news is that with modern medicine, improved surgical methods, early mobility, and energetic rehabilitation, these life-threatening complications are now less likely to occur.

Fracture of the Wrist

The forearm consists of two bones, the radius and the ulna. Fracture of the lower part of the radius near the wrist, called Colles' fracture, is most common. Bone ends are "set" back into place and immobilized with a plaster cast or splint. Follow your doctor's advice regarding use of the hand and arm during the period of healing, keeping in mind that your goal is a return of normal function. In general, exercises and light activities that promote movement of the hand, fingers, and elbow, without generating motion at the fracture site, aid healing and prevent atrophy and usually are encouraged. A sling is useful to reduce swelling and offset the weight of a cast, but should be removed frequently for range-of-motion exercises to prevent shoulder stiffness. After the cast or splint is removed, the arm will feel weak and stiff at first. Strength and function will return with normal movement. Some joint stiffness and achy pain may persist or return and may even become a predictor of weather changes.

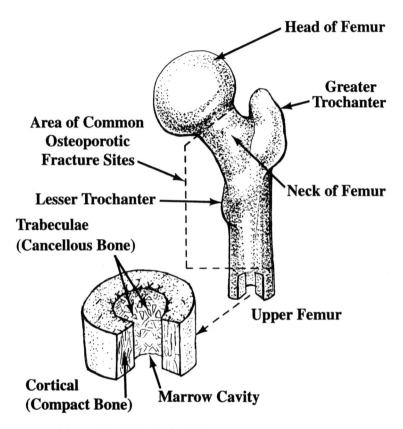

Head of Femur

Greater Trochanter

Area of Common Osteoporotic Fracture Sites

Neck of Femur

Lesser Trochanter

Trabeculae (Cancellous Bone)

Upper Femur

Cortical (Compact Bone)

Marrow Cavity

Magnified Wedge of Femur

A fracture means not only a broken bone but a break in one's daily routine and lifestyle. The transition from self-sufficiency to dependency is hard to adjust to even temporarily. Recovery, too, means more than allowing time for bone to heal. It involves giant effort and iron will. For those who no longer can care for themselves, an attitude of despair provides an added roadblock to recovery. However, if a fracture receives prompt attention, if treatment is correct and conscientious, and if rehabilitation is well designed and followed in a determined manner, the outlook for complete recovery is good in most cases.

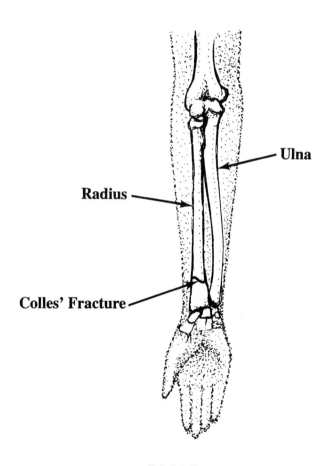

Right Forearm

18

FRACTURES OF THE SPINAL VERTEBRAE

Anyone who has osteoporosis and leads a normal active life probably will experience compression fractures of the vertebrae. Most occur after age sixty, eight times more often in women than men. We can best preserve our spine if we understand how it works.

The backbone is ingeniously designed to protect the spinal cord, support the entire body, and enable movement. It includes 24 bones stacked like doughnuts with shock-absorbing cartilage discs sandwiched between. Bones differ slightly, but all are mainly trabecular bone with a thin outer shell of cortical bone. Each has a marshmallow-shaped vertebral body in front, wing-like spikes extending to each side, and a spinous process that juts backward. Ligaments, tendons, and muscles attach to these bony prominences, fastening everything together into a remarkable functioning framework.

The spine is shaped like a shallow "S." Beneath the concave curve of seven cervical vertebrae, 12 thoracic vertebrae curve outward, each attached to a pair of ribs. The next five lumbar vertebrae compose the low back. Fused vertebrae form the sacrum and coccyx. An exaggeration of the normal curve in the thoracic area is called ky*phosis*; in the lumbar area, *lordosis*.

A healthy backbone can withstand thousands of pounds of pressure; one that is weakened by osteoporosis cannot. Most fractures occur at points of greatest stress: the weight-bearing thoracic and lumbar areas, the thoracolumbar junction where they meet, and the apex of the thoracic curve. Compression fractures may be caused by trauma, disease, or misuse, but in an osteoporotic spine they usually result from normal motions—bending, lifting, coughing, sneezing. Cracks may form. Usually the thin shell of the vertebral body gives way and weakened trabecular bone simply collapses, crushed like a marshmallow, more toward the front where the force is greatest.

As bone wedges, curving the body forward, deformity grows. Discs that absorb the jolts and jarring of strenuous actions degenerate over time, sometimes permitting painful contact of bone on bone.

Kyphosis may so compress the chest that breathing, swallowing, and cardiac difficulties result. Eventually the rib cage may rest on the hip bones, causing extreme distress. Although rare, crushed vertebrae can pinch nerves; *numbness, tingling, or weakness in the legs, pain radiating to a leg, or loss of bowel or bladder control require immediate medical attention.*

Pain, aggravated by movement, is the chief symptom of fracture. It usually is confirmed by an X ray. Pain usually is localized and often severe, but it may be mild or even absent. Intermittent or chronic dull backache may be the only hint of multiple microfractures until deformity provides undeniable testimony.

Your doctor will prescribe treatment designed to relieve pain, muscle spasm, and inflammation. Some degree of bed rest, either at home or in a hospital, may be necessary for a few days or weeks until pain subsides and healing begins. Medications reduce pain and inflammation. Warm moist compresses or a dry or moist heating pad (low to moderate setting) applied for 20 to 30 minute periods several times a day may provide comfort. (Do not use if you have diabetes or other conditions that cause decreased sensitivity to heat and could result in burns.) Gentle massage may ease muscle spasm. Pillows provide welcome support. Whatever position is most comfortable can be assumed during acute pain; a pillow under the knees eases tension. However, the spine should be kept as straight as possible when tolerated. An orthopedic garment, most helpful when standing up, also can be worn in bed for support when moving and turning.

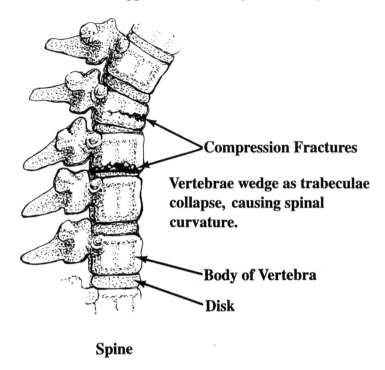

Compression Fractures

Vertebrae wedge as trabeculae collapse, causing spinal curvature.

Body of Vertebra

Disk

Spine

Pain usually tapers and subsides after a few weeks. A properly fitted brace or corset will limit motion; protect, support, and immobilize the spine; serve as a reminder to stand tall; and allow one to get out of bed and walk sooner.

Following an initial period of bed rest, with an orthopedic support in place, activity is gradually increased. As muscles weakened by inactivity brace to protect the fracture site, posture may grow increasingly unbalanced. Muscles, tendons, and ligaments may be abnormally stressed or become shorter as a result of altered gait. If the spine is unbalanced by altered body form and faulty body mechanics (Key 25), pain may become chronic and deformity may result or increase. A sound rehabilitation program will provide therapy to correct posture and enable maximum recovery.

Physical and occupational therapists teach:

- Exercises to strengthen muscles; introduction of weight-bearing exercises
- Use of assistive aids to enable mobility and a gradual return to activities of daily living
- How to identify and manage factors that predispose to falls
- Proper posture and body mechanics

Ideally, many of these measures are understood and applied before fractures occur.

Therapists are in a unique position to influence and educate. Because they spend periods of time with patients, they have ample opportunity to spot problems and anticipate and meet individual needs. They get to know their patients well, their living arrangements and lifestyles, and even meet and work with family members who will be involved with care. This close, informal relationship puts the patient at ease, more apt to share feelings and fears. A therapist has time to listen, answer questions, allay concerns, and help solve problems. With a helpful, calm attitude, a therapist can instill confidence, promote body awareness, foster a general sense of well-being, and nurture a positive self-image. Usually it is the therapist who convinces patients of the importance of rehabilitation, encouraging, challenging, and nudging them to commitment to a sometimes difficult and tedious task.

Recovery takes time and effort—it doesn't happen overnight and no one can do it for you. Your health care professionals, family, and friends are there to support you. But it's up to you to take charge so you can get back into the swing of things, back to work, and back to doing the things you want to do and enjoy doing.

19

ANALGESIC MEDICATIONS

Whether it is the sudden, excruciating pain of a new fracture or the chronic, aching back pain from old ones that limit movement and deny sleep, pain is often an unwelcome associate of osteoporosis. Pain is our body's distress signal, warning that all is not well. It is a subjective blend of feelings, sensations, and responses that exists whenever and wherever the person experiencing it says it does. When pain is well managed, we are physically comfortable, mentally satisfied, and emotionally at ease. Main strategies of pain management employ various physical comfort measures (Key 20), relaxation techniques (Key 21), and *analgesics*, that is, drugs that relieve pain. This Key examines the role of *narcotic* and nonnarcotic analgesics.

Pain is classified as acute or chronic. Acute pain is intense, short-term, and reversible, for example, pain that follows surgery or a fracture. Chronic pain continues for more than six months. It can be constant or intermittent and may change in intensity, but it is a lifelong companion.

The use of drugs to manage and control pain must be prudent, ideally providing temporary relief until comfort can be achieved by other means. Always take all medications exactly as directed. If pain persists longer than 48 hours, returns, gets worse, or is different from previous pain, contact your doctor.

Narcotic analgesics: These drugs block pain signals within the brain and spinal cord, relieving pain and altering consciousness. Most narcotic analgesics derive from opium, produce tolerance, and are habit-forming. However, when used to relieve moderate to severe pain appropriately, that is, *the smallest effective dose used for the shortest period necessary,* there is scant chance of addiction. However, precautions must be taken to safeguard against hazards posed by other side effects, which may include depressed breathing, drowsiness, confusion, a drop in blood pressure, constipation, nausea, euphoria, depression, and psychotic behavior. Older adults tend to be more sensitive to effects and side effects, and narcotic drugs must be used with caution. Smaller doses usually are adequate for pain relief. Examples of narcotic analgesics are morphine, meperidine, and codeine. *Morphine*, a powerful analgesic, is the drug of choice for severe pain. Dosage often is reduced in the elderly, especially because it greatly depresses respiration. *Meperidine* (Demerol) relieves moderate to severe pain and is used to ease anxiety before surgery. Side effects include drowsiness, dizziness, nausea, disorientation, and respiratory and circulatory depression. It should be used with caution for anyone who has asthma or impaired kidney or liver function. *Codeine* is used for milder pain, often in combination with aspirin (Emperin Number 3) or acetaminophen (Tylenol Number 3), in which case a smaller dose can be given, reducing side effects. Constipation can be a major problem. Add fruit juice and fiber to your diet, increase fluids, and get plenty of exercise if possible.

Nonnarcotic analgesics: These drugs (except acetaminophen) block nerve endings at the site of the pain. Acetaminophen blocks pain impulses at both peripheral and central nervous system levels. Nonnarcotic analgesics are less powerful, do not cause dependence, and are used to relieve mild to moderate pain. Some also reduce inflammation and are called nonsteroidal anti-inflammatory drugs (NSAIDS). Examples of nonnarcotic analgesics are acetaminophen and the NSAIDS aspirin and ibuprofen. Common side effects of nonnarcotic analgesics are indigestion, stomach ulcers, headache, and kidney or liver problems. Taking these medications with food or a full glass of milk or water reduces problems related to stomach irritation. Report bloody vomit, urine, or black stools to your doctor. *Acetaminophen* is as effective as codeine and is the preferred analgesic for noninflammatory pain. It has few side effects but long-term, high-dose use can lead to liver damage. It should be used with caution in persons with kidney or liver disease; alcohol abuse may increase its toxic potential. *Aspirin* (acetylsalicylic acid) is least expensive, as effective as codeine in pain relief, and is most effective for pain associated with inflammation. Because it is a staple in most households, we tend to discount potential hazards. Side effects include nausea, heartburn, and, most serious, gastrointestinal bleeding. Buffered or coated forms reduce gastrointestinal irritation. Aspirin should not be used by persons with bleeding disorders or those who are taking anticoagulant or ulcer-producing drugs, such as corticosteroids. *Ibuprofen* (Motrin, Advil, Nuprin) is one of many "new" NSAIDS. All are more costly and less effective than aspirin in treating inflammatory conditions, but most have a lower incidence of gastrointestinal side effects. The therapeutic effect may be delayed for two to three weeks.

Analgesic ointments and liniments: These preparations, applied topically to intact skin, may provide a soothing effect and temporary relief of minor muscle pain and stiffness by counterirritation and by improving circulation of blood to the part. Gentle massage of the aching area may enhance action by further stimulation. Examples include Ben-Gay, Eucalyptamint, and Tiger Balm.

Adjuvant Medications: Substances such as muscle relaxants and antidepressants are not analgesics, but they enhance, assist, or reinforce other strategies of pain management.

Older individuals often are stereotyped as chronic complainers of aches and pains. In fact, athough they usually have more reasons to complain, unless pain is severe, many elderly persons do not complain at all, fearing drug addiction or accepting pain as a natural part of aging. Pain is an abnormal circumstance that no one need endure. Failure to manage it can increase its intensity and its impact, crippling the body, the mind, the emotions, and the spirit.

20

PHYSICAL COMFORT MEASURES

The acute pain of a fracture can be relieved with analgesics, but what about the chronic pain that too often remains? It is difficult to be cheerful and optimistic when you are hurting. Chronic pain can be exhausting and debilitating. It also can be a blessing if it prompts action that brings relief. Discuss comfort measures with your doctor. You may be referred to a physiatrist, physical or occupational therapist, nurse, or pain specialist for further assessment of your needs and for help to manage chronic pain. Pain can and must be controlled. If it is not, then pain takes control and dictates the boundaries of your life. This Key will discuss transcutaneous electrical nerve stimulation, *acupuncture*, and the use of cold and heat, including diathermy and ultrasound.

The gate theory helps to explain why many of these methods work. Pain impulses travel along nerve fibers and pass through the spinal cord to the brain. In the gate theory, pain impulses are blocked before they reach the brain; the gate is closed, so to speak. Gate-closing nerve clusters are activated by touch, electrical current, and auditory or other stimuli. The gate also can be closed from above. *Endorphins*, the body's natural opiates, are released by nerve cells in the brain. Once activated, they circulate an analgesic effect through blood and spinal fluid.

Transcutaneous Electrical Nerve Stimulation (TENS): This method uses electrical currents to stimulate nerves to close the gate, blocking transmission of pain impulses to the brain. The battery-operated TENS unit, the size of a paging device, sends mild currents through electrodes, producing a slight tingling or vibrating sensation. If a trial period brings pain relief, a physical therapist or trained nurse can teach you how to use the unit so you can manage your own pain. Follow prescribed settings and electrode placements. Notify your doctor if pain worsens or develops in another area. This technique should not be used in individuals who are pregnant or have pacemakers. Insurance covers 80 percent of the cost of rental or purchase of a unit.

Acupuncture: This method uses the same principle as electric stimulation. The acupuncture therapist inserts thin needles into the skin in points near clusters of nerve endings, stimulating nerves to close the gate. Local needling also may trigger the release of endorphins. You may feel warmth, pinpricks, or stinging sensations. After insertion, the therapist stimulates needles electrically or by manual twirling. Acupuncture should be avoided in individuals with immunodeficiency or bleeding disorders and used with caution in persons with pacemakers. Acupuncture is safe if performed correctly, and effective in some cases. If you are considering this technique, ask your doctor to recommend a reliable practitioner.

Acupressure: In this method, thumbs, fingers, or the palm of the hand are used to apply pressure to the nerve cluster points.

Heat: This technique has long been used to soothe painful body parts. Equipment may change, but the principles have not. By increasing blood flow to the area, heat indirectly provides more oxygen and nutrients to cells, speeds removal of waste products, and thereby promotes healing. Heat also raises the pain threshold of sensory nerve endings and relaxes tension in a small area.

Heat can be applied superficially in the form of hot packs, hot water bottles, heat lamps, heating pads, and aquamatic K pads. Hot baths and heated pools and whirlpools also relax muscles and promote sedation. Moist heat is especially effective. Exercise caution in all cases to avoid burns or blisters. Make sure equipment is not defective. Maintain safe temperatures, whatever you are applying. Follow your doctor's or physical therapist's orders regarding time and frequency of application. Heat usually is applied for 15 to 30 minutes, never for longer than 45 minutes. Check your skin every five minutes. Do not lie on a heating pad or fall asleep with a heating pad in place. Avoid heat or use extra caution if circulation or sensation is impaired.

Deep heat treatments, such as diathermy and ultrasound, require special equipment and licensed personnel. Diathermy penetrates the skin and fat layers to generate heat and can be focused precisely on a specific area. It is contraindicated in the presence of diminished sensation, peripheral vascular disease, blood clots, hemorrhage, or malignancy.

Ultrasound: This technique focuses high-frequency sound waves to deep structures where they are absorbed and converted to heat. Deep heat can be applied selectively to localized areas to raise the temperature and promote healing. Ultrasound increases the flexibility of damaged tissue and may be used before massage or exercise. Most people feel a slight warmth, but no discomfort. Ultrasound is covered by insurance.

Cold: This method, long used for acute pain, is now used to relieve chronic pain. Cold produces local analgesia by decreasing the number of pain impulses that reach the brain. It can be applied as a compress, an ice bag, a chemical cold pack, an aquamatic K pad, or cold immersion. You might feel cold, burning, tingling, or numb sensations. Use extreme precaution to avoid frostbite. Follow directions exactly as ordered by your doctor or physical therapist. Use a towel or cloth as a barrier next to the skin. Never apply cold treatment for more than 20 to 30 minutes and check the skin every ten minutes for blanching or mottling, indicating frostbite. Keep in mind that those who are elderly may be more insensitive to heat and cold and may sustain tissue injury without being aware that it is occurring. Cold is contraindicated in persons with peripheral vascular disease or cold allergy, or when skin has been damaged by frostbite.

21

RELAXATION TECHNIQUES

Pain sometimes can be relieved by "mind-over-matter" relaxation techniques. In fact, the gate theory (Key 20) also suggests that attention span, the power of suggestion, anxiety, past experiences, and other brain processes are tapped for pain control. This Key will discuss briefly the use of meditation, imagery, *hypnosis*, *biofeedback*, therapeutic touch, distraction, and laughter to promote comfort. The success of these techniques will depend to a great extent on a person's commitment to them. They are safe for almost everyone and offer an opportunity for people to take an active role in the management of their own pain, a great advantage. Increased sensitivity to our own bodies and the knowledge that we have the power within us to alter our responses is itself a worthwhile benefit.

Some relaxation techniques can be done with minimal instruction. Try these comfort breaks. Take a deep breath, inhaling slowly. Close your eyes and imagine pleasant thoughts. Now slowly push all of the air out of your lungs, exhaling pain and tension. Smile. Repeat at intervals throughout the day to ease pain and anxiety and to reinforce your sense of control. Selective tightening and relaxing of muscle groups, starting at your feet, refocuses attention and often relieves even moderate pain. A variety of video and audio tapes that teach relaxation techniques and offer guided imagery are available (sometimes at your local library). Ask your doctor, nurse, or therapist to recommend what is best.

Some techniques require more training and practice or the assistance of someone trained, for example, in the arts of zen or yoga. Instructors should be reputable experts in the field. Be sure that you understand the program and are convinced of benefits before you join. Again, ask for a professional referral.

Meditation: This technique uses controlled breathing and concentration on a single phrase or object to induce relaxation and focus attention away from the pain. Because the brain only can concentrate on one item at a time, pain fades as the central focus becomes stronger.

Imagery: This technique calls forth images of happy, calming circumstances to replace painful feelings and stressful situations. If you visualize yourself pain-free, perhaps walking in a sun-spattered autumn woods, you can alter your body's response to pain.

Hypnosis: This method also can relieve pain by altering pain perception. A daydream is self-hypnosis in its mildest form. Some people can put themselves into a trance and use posthypnotic suggestion to reduce pain and anxiety. Formal hypnosis requires the services of a trained hypnotist.

Biofeedback: This method provides information about what our bodies are doing. Some people can learn to change and control body activities if they know what responses are taking place. A biofeedback machine indicates when muscles are tense, the heart is racing, or the skin is cold. With controlled breathing and muscle relaxing imagery, individuals are able to slow their heart rate or warm their skin, perhaps envisioning themselves soaking in fragrant, warm bathwater.

Therapeutic touch: This technique may relieve pain for reasons not exactly clear and possibly related to endorphin release. Whether it is the "laying on of hands," gentle massage, fingers brushing a cheek, a hand stroking the brow, or arms cradling a loved one, caring touch eases pain and promotes comfort and healing.

Distraction: This technique is an effective pain reliever, familiar to all. Boredom and monotony focus attention on our discomfort and discontent. An absorbing novel can shut out the world and the pain along with it, at least for a while. A pet or a game of cards also will take your mind off of your pain.

Television can offer hours of pleasant distraction. Paging through a picture album, pain is pushed out of conscious awareness as your mind fills with warm memories. An upbeat conversation lifts both spirits and pain. On the other hand, lengthy, disturbing conversation makes you feel more exhausted and uncomfortable than ever. Sleep and rest are very important. Frequent short naps or rest periods increase pain tolerance. Soft, soothing music or audio relaxation tapes work because endorphins are released by auditory stimulation.

Laughter: This is an especially powerful analgesic. Several years ago, Norman Cousins, author of *Anatomy of an Illness*, was suffering from a painful, debilitating, life-threatening disease. When his situation seemed hopeless, he transferred from the stark hospital environment to a pleasant hotel room and self-prescribed laughter, delivered by Marx Brothers films and "Candid Camera" replays. He found that each ten-minute "dose" of laughter resulted in at least two hours of pain-free sleep. Cousins focused attention on the benefit of belly laughs, and studies have since verified their healing power.

Pain management and rehabilitation programs: These instructional methods are becoming more prevalent as chronic pain is gaining recognition as a serious health threat. Individuals who are not able to manage disabling pain with their own doctor's help may be referred to specialists. Doctors, nurses, therapists, psychologists, and social workers work together to provide an interdisciplinary approach to pain, focusing on nondrug strategies. Services are offered in inpatient and outpatient settings.

When all else failed, Cousins adopted a creative approach to regain control of his health. Using a combination of approaches outlined in Keys 19–21, you too can gain control over pain.

22

CALCIUM SUPPLEMENTS

A controversial outcome of increased publicity about osteoporosis is that it became trendy to take calcium supplements. Calcium was the "gold" of the 80s and the rush was on. Plain old-fashioned yogurt reappeared in multiple colors, flavors, and consistencies. Antacid manufacturers switched their pitch to hype the calcium content of their products. Cereals boosted calcium content and publicized its bone-building capabilities. Armed with reports that calcium would halt crippling effects of osteoporosis, older women led the charge. Many took costly supplements without questioning possible hazards. The number of calcium preparations multiplied. Sales rose from $50 million to $250 million a year.

The dust has settled, but there is still a need to sort fact from misinformation in order to manage calcium supplements judiciously. Although it is true, for example, that calcium plays a vital role in reducing bone loss, other factors, especially estrogen, are involved. For example, a calcium supplement frequently is prescribed at the beginning of menopause *along with estrogen*. Calcium alone cannot halt the rapid bone resorption that women typically experience during this period. A supplement also is prescribed when there is a deficiency, such as in cases of the bone disorders osteomalacia and rickets. New studies indicate adequate calcium may help ward off gum disease, high blood pressure, and colon cancer. Who should take supplements? Which are best?

It is best to get vitamins and minerals from the foods we eat and drink, but it is not always possible. A staggering 42 percent of all Americans take in less than 70 percent of the recommended daily allowance of calcium. Key 29 explains how to calculate your calcium needs. If you have attempted to meet those needs by increasing the calcium in your diet and still fall short, you can make up the difference with a calcium supplement.

A calcium supplement contains elemental (pure) calcium combined with other substances to form a salt. Know what to look for on labels and read them carefully. Some labels list milligrams of the salt on the front, and break it down into elemental calcium elsewhere. For example, 650 mg of calcium gluconate contains only 58 mg of elemental calcium. You would need to take 17 tablets to get 1,000 mg of calcium. *Elemental calcium is the actual calcium you receive.* Ask your pharmacist for help and advice.

Sampling of Calcium Supplements*

Calcium Supplement	Salt	Elemental Calcium	Percent of Calcium
Calcium carbonate	750 mg	300 mg	40 %
Calcium citrate	950 mg	200 mg	21%
Calcium gluconate	650 mg	58 mg	9%
Calcium lactate	650 mg	84 mg	13%
Tricalcium phosphate	800 mg	304 mg	39%
Dicalcium phosphate	500 mg	115 mg	29%

* Dosage is measured in milligrams per tablet. Additional forms and dosages are available.

There are other factors to consider. Cost varies broadly. A generic brand that is half the price of an advertised equivalent may be just as effective. On the other hand, inexpensive tablets that are so compressed they do not dissolve well are no bargain. Some forms are distasteful. Some are chewable. Calcium glubionate is a syrup preparation.

Some antacids contain calcium, others do not. Tums, the antacid tablet, is convenient, inexpensive, pleasantly flavored, and provides 200 mg of elemental calcium in 500 mg tablets. Calcium gluconate is apt to irritate the stomach.

Calcium carbonate preparations are the most concentrated and generally least expensive, but they may be poorly absorbed by older persons and are constipating. Dolomite and bone meal may be tainted with toxic metals and should be avoided. Calcium citrate is the best choice. It is absorbed best, is least irritating to the stomach, is least likely to cause formation of kidney stones, and promotes bone mineralization better than other forms.

Some calcium supplements are available only by prescription. Most are available over-the-counter. One form might suit your particular needs better than another. If you are on a special diet, are pregnant or breast-feeding, or if you are taking any other medicine, seek your doctor's advice. In fact, it is a good idea to check with your doctor before you begin using any kind of nonprescription drugs, including vitamins and minerals.

Calcium is best absorbed if taken in divided doses several times a day with meals, or within one to one and one-half hours afterwards. The presence of food in the stomach stimulates acid secretion needed to dissolve the calcium. Absorption is further aided when you drink 8 ounces of fluid with your supplement. Most preparations dissolve within 15 to 30 minutes. To check how readily a supplement dissolves, place a tablet in a half glass of vinegar. Stir occassionally. If the tablet has not disintegrated in a half hour, it is not likely to do so in your stomach either.

Side effects are not expected; however, they do occur infrequently. If you experience constipation, diarrhea, drowsiness, headache, appetite loss, dry mouth or weakness, inform your doctor right away. Experts have developed *Recommended Dietary Allowances* (RDAs) of calcium to use as general guidelines for various age groups. Do not exceed the RDA of 1,500 mg of calcium. Excess blood calcium (hypercalcemia) can form into stones in the kidneys, causing severe pain and possible kidney damage. This is especially true if a person is dehydrated, has poor renal function, or is taking thiazide diuretics, which limit calcium excretion. Kidney stones do not usually develop unless excess calcium is taken with large amounts of vitamin D by persons susceptible to their formation. If you have a condition that interferes with calcium balance, or are taking certain medications, your doctor will advise you of how much calcium it is safe for you to take. Unless otherwise advised, follow these general guidelines:

- Get your RDA of vitamin D.
- Drink 10 to 12 glasses of fluids daily, 8 of them water.
- Take syrup preparations just before meals for better absorption.
- Chew chewable tablets before swallowing for best absorption.
- Do not take supplements within one to two hours of oral medications.
- Eat foods that are high in fiber to aid digestion and prevent constipation.
- Avoid taking supplements with foods that contain oxalic or phytic acid or foods rich in iron or zinc because absorption is altered (Key 31).
- Do not smoke cigarettes or drink large amounts of caffeine or alcohol.

23

HORMONE REPLACEMENT THERAPY

A drop in estrogen levels due to menopause or as a result of removal or impairment of both ovaries is the single most important cause of osteoporosis and accompanying fractures. And the single most effective way to prevent and treat osteoporosis is to replace that estrogen and restore its bone-protecting advantages. Recent studies reveal the significant additional value of estrogen as a deterrent to coronary artery disease, the number one killer of women. A ten-year follow-up of the Nurses' Health Study of 48,470 postmenopausal women concluded that estrogen therapy is associated with a reduced risk of coronary heart disease and death from cardio-vascular disease (Stampfer 1991). Women treated with estrogen enjoy the following benefits:

- Elimination of the distressing symptoms of menopause
- Preservation of bone tissue throughout the skeleton
- 50 percent fewer fractures of the wrist and hip
- 90 percent fewer fractures of vertebrae
- 50 percent decrease in the risk of heart attack and cardio-vascular disease
- Lower blood levels of LDL (bad) cholesterol; higher blood levels of HDL (good) cholesterol
- Decreased tissue atrophy of the vagina and lower urinary tract
- Improved quality and joy of living

Links to cancer, which arose after estrogen had been easing the stressful symptoms of menopause for decades, have been largely discounted as researchers developed preparations that are safe for most women. Studies on the risk for breast cancer have been inconsistent. A slight increase in risk noted may be related to better education, mammogram screening, closer follow-up, and longer life spans. A woman who develops breast cancer at age seventy may, in the past, have died of a heart attack at age fifty-five. Risk of endometrial cancer is based on the fact that estrogen stimulates growth of the endometrial lining of the uterus, which, when not shed, may undergo changes that can lead to cancer. Adding progesterone to estrogen therapy eliminates any increased threat of endometrial cancer and may enhance bone-sparing benefits. Furthermore, during the careful follow-up that accompanies hormone therapy, both breast lumps and endometrial changes can be detected early and treated effectively. It is important to note that studies do not show increased risk of death from breast cancer, perhaps due to earlier detection. Indeed, death from all causes is reduced in postmenopausal women who take estrogen.

With a few exceptions, the American College of Obstetricians and Gynecologists recommends the combination of estrogen and progestin, called Hormone Replacement Therapy (HRT). Therapy should be modified for women who have liver or gallbladder disease, previous side effects from estrogen, blood clotting disorders, and unexplained vaginal bleeding. A woman who has had her uterus removed needs only estrogen. Although progestin may slightly counteract some beneficial effects of estrogen in lowering the risk of coronary artery disease, the most common form (brand name Provera) appears to have little effect on lipids. The benefits of HRT still far outweigh the risks.

Generally, HRT should begin as soon after the onset of menopause as possible. In addition to the rapid rate of bone loss that normally occurs during the first few years, for one third of postmenopausal women bone loss is extreme—3 to 5 percent a year during the first four to seven years. Treatment begun at a later stage slows bone loss but cannot erase the fracture risk to bones already compromised. Nor will it clear arteries that are plugged by plaque from LDL cholesterol.

The minimum dose of oral estrogen needed to prevent bone loss is extremely low, 0.625 mg of conjugated estrogen, the most commonly used form, or its equivalent, daily. Women whose ovaries are removed before menopause usually begin with larger doses, which are then modified for long-term benefits. (A woman who needs to have her uterus removed should retain her ovaries unless there is a medical reason to remove them. The possible exception is someone with a strong family history of ovarian cancer.) The dosage necessary for bone-protecting effects of other forms of estrogen—vaginal cream, injections, skin patches—are yet unknown. Presently, oral estrogen is the only drug approved by the FDA for both prevention and treatment of osteoporosis. The cost is $200 to $300 per year.

Estrogen may be given on a cyclic basis, with progesterone added during part of each month. This method typically produces light monthly uterine bleeding. Or, low doses of both hormones may be given daily. After an initial period of spotting during the first few months, this method usually eliminates the monthly bleeding that women find troublesome. Other regimens are possible.

If you are entering the menopausal period, a gynecologist who specializes in the health care of women is best suited to offer counsel and treatment and answer your questions and concerns regarding HRT. Together, weigh personal benefits and risks—of osteoporosis, heart disease, cancer—and decide on the best course of treatment for *you*. Faith in your doctor is important. Faith in your own ability to understand and be part of decision making is equally important.

Close monitoring and proper management are essential. You should have an annual physical examination, including a pelvic examination and Pap test (a smear swabbed from the cervix of the uterus is examined for abnormal cells), as well as a pretreatment and a yearly mammogram (X ray of the breasts). An endometrial sampling may be done. If there is any question about treatment, a bone mass measurement should be done to aid decision making. Report unexpected uterine bleeding immediately. Check your breasts for lumps monthly. Watch your calcium intake. Less estrogen is needed if you consume adequate amounts. Drink ample fluids. Get plenty of exercise to stimulate blood circulation, especially in your legs.

Substantial evidence of the benefits of estrogen exists from scores of studies, yet it remains a somewhat controversial issue. Research is ongoing. Further clinical studies will expand knowledge regarding its effect on women who already have established coronary artery disease; the effect of adding progestin, from which women are most likely to benefit; and other areas.

However, it is clear that estrogen deters the deadly course of osteoporosis and coronary artery disease, two diseases that claim the lives of millions of women. The majority of women will not get cancer; the majority of women will die from the complications of osteoporosis and heart disease. Unless there is evidence of active, estrogen-dependent cancer, most experts agree that estrogen replacement should begin as soon as possible after menopause and should continue indefinitely.

24

DRUG THERAPY

Drug treatment regimens fall into two categories: those that *inhibit* bone resorption (stabilizing bone mass at its present level) and those that *stimulate* bone formation (adding to the bone mass that already is there). Some drugs do both, or are used in combination. Adequate calcium and vitamin D intake is essential for maximum effectiveness of all drug therapy.

Most drugs are of the *antiresorptive* type: estrogen, calcitonin, the bisphosphonates, and calcium. Estrogen and calcium already have been discussed. Anabolic steroids, calcitriol (vitamin D), and progestin analogs also are antiresorptive, but may have some effect on bone formation. Presently only estrogen and synthetic salmon calcitonin have FDA approval for osteoporosis treatment. However, doctors may prescribe drugs that are approved for another use.

Sodium fluoride, a fragment of parathormone, and various growth factors *stimulate bone formation.* These drugs are undergoing extensive testing and one day may become the dominant treatment for established osteoporosis.

Calcitonin: This thyroid hormone acts directly through receptors in osteoclasts, inhibiting their bone resorption activity and thus reducing bone loss. Studies indicate a small increase in total body calcium and in bone mass in the spine and radius, decreased bone loss in the spine, hip, and total skeleton in postmenopausal women with spinal fractures, and faster healing after hip fractures. There is some evidence that the initial increase in bone mass tapers after a few years. Calcitonin may also relieve back pain caused by spinal fractures, a welcome advantage.

Because oral forms are inactivated by gastrointestinal secretions, calcitonin is administered by injection. Cost is between $2,000 and $3,000 per year. Side effects such as flushing and nausea occur in 10 to 20 percent of cases but are not sufficient to stop treatment. Nasal sprays, presently used only in research, may soon offer an alternative to injections, with the added advantage of reducing side effects. Calcitonin is most often used for severe osteoporosis, but also may be beneficial in glucocorticoid-induced osteoporosis, and as an alternative preventive treatment in postmenopausal osteoporosis for women who do not take estrogens.

Bisphosphonates: These drugs reduce bone resorption and prevent bone loss and vertebral fractures, especially in postmenopausal and glucocorticoid-induced osteoporosis. Questions remain regarding nonvertebral fractures, bone strength, long-term skeletal impact, and specifics regarding dosage and administration. Side effects are minor for most preparations.

A two-year American study (Watts et al. 1990) of 429 postmenopausal women with osteoporotic fractures of the vertebrae tested *etidronate*, a first generation bisphosphonate that has been used for over ten years to treat Paget's disease of the bone. Those who were treated alternately with etidronate to slow bone resorption and prevent further vertebral collapse, and calcium to aid bone formation, had an average increase of 5 percent in bone mass and 50 percent fewer new fractures than the control group. The cost of treatment is $200 to $300 per year.

Sodium fluoride: This chemical element that dentists have been using for years to strengthen teeth, may one day do the same for bones. Fluoride increases spinal bone mass by increasing the number of osteoblasts, thus stimulating bone formation. Its effect on fracture incidence is controversial and might be dose dependent. There is some concern that stress fractures may result from therapy.

Preparations used in early studies revealed troublesome side effects, including pain in the large joints of the lower extremities in 25 to 40 percent of patients, and gastrointestinal distress in 25 to 30 percent (pain, nausea, vomiting, and, rarely, hemorrhage). These symptoms have been largely reduced in most cases by lower, equally effective doses of coated or slow-release preparations, or by interrupted therapy.

Fluoride is a unique agent that increases bone mass substantially in 70 percent of patients treated. Long-term fluoride and calcium therapy presently is established treatment in Europe. However, conflicting findings and uncertainties regarding skeletal complications have put this potent bone builder on the back burner for now. It remains an experimental agent, used for clinical research only.

Anabolic steroids: These are synthetic derivations of the male hormone, testosterone. They appear to inhibit bone resorption and increase bone formation. Studies have shown improvement in spinal, wrist, and total skeletal bone mass over two-year periods, but no evidence of reduced fractures. Long-term use is limited by side effects, which may include sodium and fluid retention, masculinizing effects, and impaired liver function. Altered lipid metabolism may cause an increase in low-density lipoproteins, which promote the harmful buildup of fatty deposits in blood vessels that is associated with atherosclerosis and coronary artery disease.

Studies show that intermittent administration of parathormone stimulates osteoblast activity and increases total bone mass. Insulin-like growth factors may help regulate bone turnover; research on growth factors has uncovered optimistic findings. There is evidence that androgens stimulate bone formation. Calcitriol is thought to hinder the bone-resorbing action of parathormone and stimulate bone formation. A comprehensive study reported a reduced number of vertebral compression fractures with no significant side effects in women with postmenopausal osteoporosis. Other studies have had conflicting results and note that decreased fracture incidence may be due to the ability of vitamin D to increase calcium absorption. Modest increases in bone density occur, suggesting a major role of calcitriol in prevention and justifying further studies as well as studies using other vitamin D analogs.

At the present time, the medicine chest of drug therapy yields promising potions. The value of estrogen and calcitonin is recognized. Bisphosphonates show great potential as inhibitors of bone resorption. They are available in oral form, are moderate in cost, are safe when used intermittently, and are potentially effective, especially in cases of established osteoporosis. Newer, more potent bisphosphonates are being tested for future use for both treatment and prevention. Sodium fluoride stimulates bone formation and increases density, but unfortunately the quality of bone produced may be inferior. In the search for safe, affordable, effective treatments, perhaps even cure, studies continue on these and other agents. Drugs are tested for bone-building and fracture-reducing properties and long-term benefits, using varying doses, preparations, techniques, and combinations. As research moves forward with increasing urgency, the future looks very bright indeed.

25

POSTURE AND BODY MECHANICS

The back needs lifelong attention for good health: good *posture*, proper exercise, and correct use, called *body mechanics*. Let's examine each point more closely.

An understanding of the force of gravity is helpful. It can be a formidable foe if you work against it.

The center of gravity of the body is in the pelvis; our feet provide the base of support. The relationship between the center of gravity in the pelvis and the base of support determines how stable we are. If either shifts, for example, if we put our weight on one leg as we reach to the side, the body becomes unbalanced. We become more stable when we lower the center of gravity, for example, by squatting. We widen our base of support by putting our feet apart.

To increase awareness of posture, the National Chiropractic Association conducted a survey judged by specialists in spinal problems. "Winners" included: Candice Bergen for most regal; George Bush for most commanding male; and Arnold Schwarzenegger for most macho. Clearly good posture projects images, such as grace, attitude, energy, and well-being.

Good posture is neither rigid nor strained; it becomes a natural and comfortable habit that enhances the health of the spine. Stand as tall as you can with your head up, shoulders back, and stomach muscles taut. You have good posture if your ears, shoulders, hips, knees, and ankles are aligned with an imaginary plumb line stretched vertically next to your body. When the curves of our spine are in correct position, our body is balanced, weight is distributed evenly throughout the vertebrae and discs, and our joints suffer the least amount of strain.

The spine is supported by muscles of the back and abdomen. Movement disorders—chronic, repetitive movements that put undue stress and strain on the spine and surrounding tissue—and uneven gait, exaggerated over time—can lead to serious problems. Muscles weakened by disease, poor posture, obesity, disuse, or misuse, do not supply adequate support. As we get older, our posture shifts slightly, away from "correct." Muscle strain, stiffness, pain, fatigue, and even deformity may result. However, if our muscles are strong from exercise that is done properly and regularly, they will hold our body parts in good alignment, help resist the power of gravity to cause bowed legs, swayed backs, and stooped shoulders; and make us less vulnerable to strain and injury. And the stronger the back muscles, the denser will be the bones in the spine.

Like the supporting framework of a building, there is a correct relationship among all parts of our skeleton. Unlike the framework of a building, our bodies are dynamic. Parts constantly change both position and relationship as we stand, sit, and move about. We practice good body mechanics when we distribute our weight and our work load properly. Follow these guidelines:

Lifting: Lifting even light objects improperly puts a great strain on your back and can cause injury. Modify daily activities to avoid twisting or bending forward at the waist, movements that put pressure on the vertebrae. Instead of bending over to lift objects from the floor, bend your knees, hold the object close to your body, and tighten your stomach muscles. Keep your back straight and let your legs and shoulders do the work. Never twist and lift at the same time; turn your feet instead. If the object is heavy, or if you have to lift it higher than your waist, get help. Overloading the spine when bones are compromised by osteoporosis invites crush fractures.

Sitting: Chairs you sink into and hardly can get out of may feel comfortable but they put pressure on the spine, stretch ligaments, and cause muscle fatigue. An ideal chair provides firm support for your back and thighs and positions your knees level with your hips and your feet flat on the floor. Armrests help you get up and down by using arm muscles instead of your back. Sit close to your work so you don't need to lean over. Never hold your neck in a twisted position or prop a phone in the crook of your neck. Correct posture is especially important if you spend a great deal of time in a chair or wheelchair. Use small pillows for back support.

Standing: Sitting actually is more stressful to the back, but we seem to get more tired standing up. When standing, shift your weight, alternately resting one foot on a shelf or stool. If you sit or stand for long periods of time, walk around at least every hour. Keep your blood circulating with foot exercises: wriggle your toes, step in place.

Lying/sleeping: A good position for sleep is on your side or back with your knees slightly bent. A pillow under your neck should support your head and keep it level but not force it forward. Keep small pillows handy to support your back. A firm mattress or a bedboard under a sagging mattress also supports the spine and aids good posture. Never sleep in a chair. Don't lie on the sofa or in bed and read with your head propped sharply against the armrest or headboard.

It is always important to take proper care of our back, but a backbone that is weakened by osteoporosis requires special care. Those who already have sustained fractures may have further restrictions, for example, to avoid heavy lifting. Your doctor will suggest added precautions you should take. However, we can all develop posture awareness. Even when standing tall no longer is possible, we can exercise to strengthen muscles of support and remind ourselves to stand and walk as straight as we are able. Thereby, we can enhance comfort and minimize the disabling and disfiguring effects of osteoporosis.

26

ESTABLISHING A PROGRAM OF MAXIMUM MANAGEMENT

So far this book has examined the broad picture of a major health problem and to a microscopic view of bone itself. You may believe you know all that you need to—and more. "As I extinguish 65 candles on my birthday cake, do I really want to know that my chances of breaking a bone are now one in three?" you might ask. Or, "If I have the misfortune to break a hip, am I as likely to end up dead or in a nursing home as I am to recover?" Statistics are admittedly stark. They are not meant to overwhelm, but rather to impress you with the seriousness of osteoporosis and to instill in you the determination to resist it with every means available and medically recommended.

A 1991 Gallup poll conducted for the National Osteoporosis Foundation affirmed that American women are dangerously ignorant of the gravity of osteoporosis. The peril lies in the fracture potential, yet over 80 percent of those surveyed did not make the connection among the 300,000 hip, 500,000 spinal, and 200,000 wrist fractures and osteoporosis. Although fewer than 60 percent of respondents could identify major risk factors, it is heartening to find that almost all correctly named poor nutrition and two thirds correctly cited lack of exercise as risk factors. You have a running start if you are informed. The next section will demonstrate how to outsmart osteoporosis with diet and exercise.

Sound nutrition and exercise that promotes strength, flexibility, and endurance are our most effective shields, benefiting even seriously advanced osteoporosis. It helps us look and feel brighter, heal faster, and think more clearly. We also live longer and happier and reduce the risk of developing heart disease, high blood pressure, and diabetes. If a potion could retard aging, protect our blood vessels, fire us with energy, end insomnia, ease tension, trim our body, step up mobility, and improve our sex life, we'd mortgage our house to get it. Exercise is just such a potion, the closest we can get to the fountain of youth.

Osteoporosis is preventable if bone loss has not yet occurred or if it is detected early and managed efficiently. Mindful of your risk factors, seek medical care and begin today to make healthy lifestyle changes. There is much we can do for ourselves to achieve the goal of vigorous longevity.

Management Before Osteoporosis Is Detectable
(through about age forty)

Goals:
- Identify/reduce risk factors.
- Develop positive lifestyle habits.
- Build/maintain bone density.

Actions:
- Become informed regarding positive lifestyle.
  Read books and other health literature.
  Attend classes.
  Talk to your doctor, nurse, or other health professionals.
- Calculate your risk factors; work to eliminate them.
- Quit smoking; limit caffeine and alcohol intake.
- Eat a nutritionally balanced, calcium-rich diet.
- Exercise regularly to increase/maintain flexibility, strength, endurance, and bone mass. Check with your doctor before beginning an exercise program.
- Take medications only as needed and exactly as prescribed.
- Follow medical advice regarding health problems.

Management to Prevent Progression of
Early Osteoporosis
(ages thirty-five through sixty)

Goals:

- Detect osteoporosis in early stages.
- Maintain bone density.
- Maintain the integrity of the skeleton—prevent fractures.

Actions:

- Become informed regarding bone density measurement, dietary supplements, weight-bearing exercise, hormone replacement therapy (HRT), and treatments available.
- Follow previous management protocol.
- Increase calcium intake as necessary to compensate for factors that hinder utilization.
- Take supplements as prescribed.
- Correct lactose intolerance, if present.
- Review your exercise program with your doctor. Consider referral to a physical therapist for an individualized regimen that stresses weight-bearing exercise.
- Minimize health problems; safeproof your environment.
- Discuss risks, benefits, and begin hormone replacement if recommended by your doctor; comply with conscientious follow-up to treatment.
- Calcitonin or any other drug therapy may be indicated.
- Reduce disruptive stress, plan fun activities/sports/socialization.
- Maintain optimum activity/function.

27

MANAGING ADVANCED OSTEOPOROSIS: A SUCCESS STORY

Anne is a sixty-five-year-old social worker. Her interests are literature, travel, and people. She lives with her sister in an apartment complex, home to people of every age and circumstance. Anne provides inspiring proof that happiness, growth, and fulfillment are not confined by a wheelchair.

On a home visit one day, Anne lifted a child onto her lap and felt a sharp pain in her lower back. The pain persisted while Anne spent a week in bed, nursing with a moist heating pad and aspirin what she thought was muscle strain. After three weeks she returned to work, moving cautiously, still feeling discomfort.

Six months later, Anne was shopping with a friend when a hearty laugh rose to a cry of anguish. Spinal X rays revealed an old wedge fracture and a new compression fracture. Anne realized from her personal history that she was at high risk for osteoporosis: a slight, white woman who drank coffee instead of milk, smoked heavily most of her life (she recently stopped), and shunned exercise. A physical examination, laboratory tests, and a bone scan confirmed osteoporosis. Her doctor prescribed hormone replacement, calcitonin, and analgesic medications.

Anne used her recovery time wisely. She was anxious to learn about osteoporosis, and her team of professional care providers was anxious to teach her how to manage it. A dietitian showed her how to get more calcium and vitamin D in her diet and warned her about excesses, especially her favorites, coffee and phosphorus-rich soft drinks. A physical therapist taught her body mechanics and exercises that would help ward off further fractures. She spent time with an occupational therapist in a room designed to teach patients how to adapt their home environment and modify routine daily living activities. And she learned to use a walker, a hard reality to accept. Anne went home with cervical traction, a corset, reacher and walker, instructions for daily exercises, and plans to make her apartment safe and convenient—"spine-friendly."

That was ten years ago. Anne since has suffered a broken hip and developed adult onset diabetes. Diet and exercise are critical elements of her daily life. She wears her corset most of the time. Sometimes her brace offers more support and pain relief and gives her more "breathing" space. She uses a walker for short distances, but walking is very painful; she spends most of her time in a wheelchair—never just sitting.

Anne does wheelchair exercises, including deep breathing to aerate lungs that are restricted in their ability to expand due to increasing kyphosis. Small pillows of every size and shape ease tense muscles, support posture, and relieve pressure points. Although pain is a fairly constant companion, Anne rarely needs narcotics, relying instead on an arsenal of alternate comforters: aspirin, NSAIDS, heat, TENS, relaxation tapes, Mozart, and friends. She finds swimming in warm water especially beneficial and joins a friend for swim therapy at least twice a week.

Accustomed to helping others, her most difficult adjustment was accepting outside help. At first she resisted, but as a social worker, she had seen too many homebound individuals further handicapped by rejecting help, other people, and eventually, life. As her disease progressed, Anne learned to accept meals and services from friends and neighbors, and, later on, from home care personnel.

Anne admits that it was hard to give up some activities, but she found that the spaces they occupied were filled quickly with other, often more rewarding, tasks. Lifelong interests continue, modified by her circumstances. A wheelchair tray enables her to maintain a comfortable position while writing and reading. A console phone protects her neck during endless conversations for business and pleasure. She tape records books that the local library circulates to the visually impaired. An activist for broader access to public places and transporation for the handicapped, Anne is delighted to see society increasingly facing this issue. She presently is planning a trip to New England with her sister.

By pacing activities and scheduling rest periods to avoid the pain that accompanies fatigue, Anne still is able to apply her social work skills at home. She has converted her apartment complex of strangers to a close, caring community. She coordinates day care for children and adults, welcomes newcomers, informs residents of community services to fill their needs, and matches needs with offers of help from fellow tenants. For spending money, she cares for three neighbor children after school. They love to look at her pictures and hear of places she has been. Once an avid shopper, Anne claims catalog shopping doubles enjoyment—making choices, then opening packages after she's forgotten what she's ordered. She reads extensively and is an interesting and informed conversationalist, but also a good listener. Friends enjoy her company and wise counsel. The support system provided by family and friends, along with the help and support from her extended family of professional care providers have allowed her to maintain control of her life.

For those who, like Anne, are experiencing the chronic effects of osteoporosis, seemingly unavoidable problems often are within our ability to manage and control. In some instances, you must learn to live with limitations that osteoporosis imposes. In most instances, you can improve your circumstances substantially. We wouldn't keep a child at home who needed a brace to walk, yet many adults become homebound and socially isolated because they are dependent on a walker. Tested and pushed to the limits, Anne has emerged a stronger person with a firmer grasp of the value of life. You can do the same.

Management of Advanced Osteoporosis (after age fifty
fracture/pain are present; deformity may be present)

Goals:
- Prevent further fractures/deformity.
- Maintain optimum function and independence; a significant, zestful life.
- Provide pain relief; comfort.
- Adapt psychosocial adjustment and mental growth.

Actions:
- Become informed regarding rehabilitation options, adaptive and assistive devices, drug treatments, analgesic drugs, physical and psychological comfort measures, psychosocial outlets.
- Follow previous management protocol.
- Seek immediate treatment of fracture.
- Follow rehabilitation program, including exercises prescribed by doctor/rehabilitation team.
- Comply with all treatment and follow-up for maximum benefit.
- Examine comfort measures; apply those that work.
- Consider/discuss drug therapy if advised by your doctor.
- Arrange for and accept help as needed.
- Identify psychosocial needs; accept help and counsel to meet them.
- Establish a support system; nurture relationships.

Medicine is in the miracle business. A heart transplant was as farfetched as a trip to the moon when many of us were born. A bone-building miracle may be just ahead. The miracles that matter most often are those that take place inside, as we face hard realities and rise to greater heights, not just in spite of them, but often because of them. What matters most are those miracles that we make possible by our own efforts to go for the gusto. In big and little ways, we are potters of our own future, shaping it every day for good or bad. The quality of life for each of us is in good hands—our own.

28

BASIC NUTRITION

The role of food in health and survival has been understood since time began. However, not until the late 1700s did scientists begin to link food and disease. Now connections are clear. Certain foods can harm us; others actually protect us from disease. The National Cancer Institute notes that one third of all cancer deaths are related to our diet. The National Center for Health Statistics cites poor diet as a factor in 75 percent of all deaths. We can't always avoid illness and disease, but following the best diet possible will go a long way toward preventing problems linked with them—including osteoporosis. Foods contain nourishing substances called *nutrients*. More than 50 are important to health and vitality. Adequate vitamin D, phosphorus, protein, and especially calcium are necessary to prevent osteoporosis. However, a basic knowledge of nutrition, plus good eating habits, are critical not only for the welfare of our bones, but also for overall vibrant health. Let's begin with a mini-review of nutrition.

Nutrients are divided into six classes: carbohydrates, fats, proteins, vitamins, minerals, and water. **Carbohydrates** are composed of sugars, starches, and fiber. They should be the backbone of our diet, providing 50 to 65 percent of our total calories. Sugars and starches are our main source of energy. Refined sugars are simple carbohydrates, readily absorbed. Except for a quick energy fix (and a quicker let down), *sugar* provides "empty calories," nothing but weight and tooth decay. For quick energy *plus* healthy nutrients, choose foods with natural sugars—fruits, vegetables, and milk. *Starches* are called complex carbohydrates. Their structure is more complicated and must be broken down before it can be used by the body. Starchy foods have a "fattening" reputation, but it is usually the added fat and sugar that boosts calories. Half of the calories in some breakfast cereals are sugar. A baked potato has few calories until you add a pat of butter (calories double) or cheese sauce (calories triple). The tough part of fruits, vegetables, and grains is *fiber*. It can't be digested, so it is not a nutrient. Its valuable task is to provide bulk to push food and waste through the digestive tract to maintain bowel regularity.

Fats provide concentrated energy. In the energy order, sugars digest most rapidly so they are fast energy fuels, starches are slower, and fats are slowest of all, providing a steady, even-burning fuel. Fat is stored all over our body to pad and insulate us. If we need more energy than our food and reserves furnish, our body converts stored fat. Fats also absorb vitamins and form hormones and cell membranes. Two kinds of fats are *unsaturated* and *saturated*. Unsaturated fats come from plant sources, are usually liquid at room temperature, and contain the "good" *high-density lipoprotein (HDL)* cholesterol that helps prevent heart disease. Saturated fats, on the other hand, come from animal products and tropical oils, are usually solid at room temperature, and contain the "bad" *low-density lipoprotein (LDL)* cholesterol that plugs arteries and causes cardiovascular disease. Daily fat intake for adults should not exceed 30 percent of our total calories; 25 percent is preferable. No more than 10 percent of the total fat intake should be saturated fat.

Proteins, used to build new cells, repair damaged cells, and replace old cells that are worn out, should provide 12 to 20 percent of our total calories. Proteins are made of amino acids; eight of them are essential in our daily diet. Most animal sources contain all eight essential amino acids and are complete protein. Plant foods contain some, but not all amino acids, and are incomplete proteins. They can be combined easily for complete protein.

Vitamins and **minerals** are our safeguards; tiny amounts are absolutely vital to maintain normal metabolism. Vitamins C and B complex dissolve in water, are excreted in the urine, and must be replenished daily. Vitamins A, D, E, and K are stored in body fat. Calcium, potassium, phosphorus, iron, magnesium, zinc, fluoride, and other minerals, along with vitamins, are essential to preserve life and health. Eating a variety of foods is the best way to get all that we need.

Water composes 60 percent of our body weight and is our most essential nutrient. It is vital for all body functions and is in and around every cell. It carries oxygen and nutrients in blood and tissue fluid to cells to be burned for growth and repair, maintenance and energy production. It also removes waste products and heat. This process is called metabolism. Six to 10 cups of liquid a day (water is best) promotes efficient body functions.

Carbohydrates, proteins, fats, vitamins, and minerals provide fuel for energy and raw materials for growth and repair of tissues. Water is the medium in which all chemical reactions take place. A proper balance of these nutrients will keep us operating at top-notch efficiency. As you eat healthily, be a model and a teacher, helping and encouraging your family, friends, and especially any young people to safeguard their health with proper nutrition.

29

DAILY CALCIUM
REQUIREMENTS

Calcium is the most abundant mineral in our body. Absorbed from the food we eat, it travels through the bloodstream and circulates in the fluid that bathes every cell, activating enzymes and regulating chemical activities of cells. Without calcium, blood would not clot, our hearts would not beat, muscles would not contract, and nerves would not carry messages. Preliminary studies show that calcium also plays a significant role in lowering blood pressure in some individuals.

And calcium forms bone; 98 percent of the calcium in our body is in our bones. The other 2 percent is divided equally between teeth and the blood and soft tissues. If we do not consume enough calcium in our diet, if too little is absorbed from the intestines, or too much is excreted by the kidneys, it is withdrawn from bones for use whenever and wherever it is needed. This easy flow between blood and bones enables the body to maintain a constant blood concentration. An estimated 700 mg of calcium (found in 2⅓ cups of milk) enters and leaves the bones of an adult every day. Milk, our primary source of dietary calcium, contains 300 milligrams of calcium per cup. The National Academy of Sciences defines our Recommended Dietary Allowances (RDAs) of vitamins and minerals. A lifelong, adequate supply of calcium is a major deterrent to fractures later in life. Even a mild deficiency, extended over a period of time, is a major contributing factor for osteoporosis. Unfortunately, many Americans fall far short.

We know that bones begin life as membranes and cartilage. Hardening takes place even before a baby is born as minerals are layered to form bone. Our birth weight in calcium is about 1 ounce. Breast milk and formula can provide a **baby's RDA of 360–540 mg of calcium** (found in 1 to 2 cups of milk).

From **ages one to ten,** children run uphill at a steady pace toward the goal—peak bone mass. The skeleton grows; bones become longer, thicker, and heavier. Less than the **RDA of 800 mg of calcium** (contained in 2⅔ cups of milk) during this period of rapid growth may leave bones and teeth malformed.

During adolescence, calcium requirements increase to accommodate the dramatic growth spurt that takes place, and the body adds 1 ounce a week of new calcium. In a great push toward maturity, bones continue to grow longer, denser, and stronger as the body packs in minerals. If ever there was a time to build for the future, it is now. High bone mass at skeletal maturity is the best protection against age-related decline.

Too many adolescents never reach their goal. For **ages eleven through nineteen,** the **RDA is 1,200 mg of calcium** (found in 4 cups of milk). Unfortunately, about 35 percent of teenage boys and 87 percent of teenage girls get less than that amount. Bones that lack calcium are at a greater risk of developing osteoporosis, not only because there is less mass to begin with, but because their owners have not learned healthy eating habits along the way.

On entering adulthood, building continues at a slower pace until bone tissue has matured. Studies show that 25 to 50 percent of males and 75 percent of females between the ages of **nineteen and thirty-four** do not get the **RDA of 800 mg** (contained in 2⅔ cups of milk), much less the more appropriate **recommendation of 1,000 mg of calcium** (contained in 3⅓ cups of milk). These individuals may never reach optimal bone mass. But it's not too late. Bone formation still outpaces its removal. Although growth of the skeleton is essentially complete at about age twenty-five, an estimated 10 to 15 percent of total bone mass may be added between the ages of twenty-five and thirty-five.

Along life's path, two conditions alter calcium requirements. Menopause was discussed in Key 8. During **pregnancy and lactation** the need for calcium leaps to **1,200 to 1,600 mg** (found in 4 to 5⅓ cups of milk) to accommodate added demands of a developing baby. The body adapts somewhat. Hormone levels rise to protect bones. Calcium absorption nearly doubles. However, if there is not enough calcium to go around, Baby comes first, and Mom's bones suffer. Breast-feeding drains even more calcium than does pregnancy. A women can lose 6 percent of her bone mass nursing one child. The problem multiplies with each pregnancy, even with adequate calcium intake. If you have breast-fed several children, consider your added risk.

From a bone mass perspective, we are over the hill beginning at about age forty. Although we still can make new bone, removal begins to overtake replacement. To keep bones from diminishing, **adults** need **1,000 to 1,500 mg of calcium** (found in 3⅓ to 5 cups of milk) to help counter age-related physiological and lifestyle changes that increase the need for calcium. Adults over age forty-five consume less than half of that amount.

Recommended Dietary Allowances (RDAs) are the amounts of nutrients judged by the Food and Nutrition board of the National Academy of Sciences to be adequate to meet the needs of average healthy people. They are ample rather than minimum requirements. Based on more recent research, the National Institutes of Health advise greater amounts. Use NIH figures to calculate your RDA.

The Food and Drug Administration (FDA) averages RDA figures into four age groups, and sets the US Recommended Daily Allowances (US RDAs) which you see on food and supplement packages or on-site labels in stores. Nutritional values are expressed as percentages of the US RDA. The US RDA for calcium is based on 1,000 mg, so add a zero to the percentage to determine mg. (RDAs noted throughout this book are for average healthy adults, unless otherwise stated.)

If you need supplements, abide by these standards or take as directed by your doctor. Read labels carefully. Never take megadoses, defined as ten times the RDA. More than one third of all Americans spend $3 billion a year on vitamin and mineral supplements. If you eat a nutritionally adequate diet, they are a waste of money, unless they are needed for a specific health problem.

Recommended Daily Dietary Calcium
(1 cup of milk contains 300 mg of calcium)

Age/Condition	*RDA mg calcium	**NIH mg calcium
Infants: Birth to 6 months	360 mg	
6 months to 1 year	540 mg	
Children: 1 to 10 years	800 mg	
Adolescents: 10 to 19 years	1,200 mg	
Adults: Men and women	800 mg	1,000 mg
Women pregnant/lactating		
under 19 years	1,600 mg	
over 19 years	1,200 mg	
Women after menopause		
not taking estrogens		1,500 mg
taking estrogens		1,000 mg

* Based on Recommended Dietary Allowances, National Academy of Sciences, 1980.

** Recommendations based on research findings of the National Institutes of Health, 1984.

30

VITAMINS, MINERALS, AND BONES

Suppose our diet contains ample calcium. Can we breathe a sigh of relief, knowing our bones are safe and sound? That would be much too simple. And by now you know osteoporosis is anything but simple.

Calcium requires other "ingredients" to help produce strong, straight bones. In this Key and the next, we see how other factors—vitamins, minerals, protein, fiber, salt, lactose intolerance—enhance or hinder the utilization of calcium in relation to osteoporosis.

Vitamin D: This vitamin aids calcium absorption. Guzzling milk is of limited value if vitamin D is not there to "open the door" so calcium can enter the bloodstream. And vitamin D cannot perform the task of doorman unless the body, triggered by parathormone, converts it to an active hormonal form, calcitriol, in the liver and kidneys. Without calcitriol to aid mineral absorption, bones will not harden properly. "Soft" bones are easily bent out of shape, a condition called *rickets* in children, common until cod-liver oil, rich in vitamin D, was found to be an effective treatment. Because of the widespread use of vitamin D-fortified milk, rickets is rare today in this country. A similar condition in adults is called *osteomalacia*. It is characterized by a bone softening due to decalcification, particularly of bones in the spine, pelvis, and lower extremities. Both conditions are treated with vitamin D.

Vitamin D is manufactured when skin is exposed to sunlight. At least 15 minutes of exposure a day is recommended. In winter climates that may be impossible. Fish liver oils, fortified cereals, and dairy products are excellent substitutes. Persons who lack adequate sun exposure or dietary intake, and the elderly, who do not manufacture and use vitamin D efficiently, may need a supplement. The **RDA of vitamin D is 400 international units (IU)**. (One cup of milk provides 100 IU.) Fat-soluble, vitamin D is stored in the body and therefore may build to excess over time and can cause high blood levels of calcium, kidney stones, and actual bone loss. *Do not exceed the RDA without medical advice.*

Phosphorus: This element is part of nearly every chemical reaction and is a key element of the nucleic acids DNA and RNA that carry our hereditary genes. About 80 percent of the phosphorus in our body is in our bones and teeth. It is present in nearly all foods—meats (hamburger patty, 134 mg), eggs (one egg, 90 mg), dairy products (1 cup milk, 228 mg), poultry, fish, legumes, and whole grain cereals. A balanced diet easily provides the **800 mg RDA of phosphorus**. The average American gets twice that amount.

Like calcium, phosphorus moves in and out of bones to maintain a normal blood ratio. Too much of either mineral interferes with absorption of both. A high phosphorus intake stimulates parathormone, increasing bone resorption. Increased use of phosphate additives to processed meats, cheese, salad dressings, refrigerated baked goods, and beverages contributes significant amounts to the diet. With the popularity of soft drinks, the possible risk of bone loss to those, for example, who drink three or more sodas on a daily basis in addition to phosphorus-rich foods must be considered. (Cola-type carbonated beverages contain 52 mg of phosphorus, artificially sweetened drinks have slightly less.) To keep the calcium/phosphorus ratio in balance, avoid large amounts of phosphorus and minimal amounts of calcium.

Magnesium: This is our fourth most abundant element. It aids muscle contraction and nerve stimulation; 60 percent of the body's supply is in bones. A balanced diet will provide adequate magnesium, found in green leafy vegetables, whole grains, seafood, dried beans, milk, and nuts. Excessive amounts upset calcium and phosphorus metabolism and balance, and inhibit bone calcification. Conversely, lack of magnesium may lower blood calcium levels and impair growth. Deficiency is rare, but when it does occur, it usually is associated with alcoholism, diabetes, malabsorption, and kidney and glandular disorders.

Zinc: This element aids bone calcification and hormonal and enzyme activity—probably even memory. It is found where new bone is forming and is known to speed healing. Oysters (1 mg per oyster), liver (1 mg per ounce), milk (1 mg per cup), herring, and whole grains are good sources. The **RDA for zinc is 15 mg.** Deficiency may result in taste abnormalities, retarded growth, and dwarfism. Laxatives and phytates inhibit absorption; diuretics, cirrhosis of the liver, and alcohol abuse may increase excretion.

Sodium: Too much **sodium** increases excretion of calcium. The average American consumes 15 pounds of salt per year, many times more than the **RDA of 3,000 mg of sodium** daily. One teaspoon of salt contains 2,000 mg of sodium (table salt is 40 percent sodium). Sodium occurs naturally in many foods. Older kidneys have trouble handling excess salt and it may be retained in body tissues. This can raise blood pressure and lead to a stroke, or heart or kidney disease. How to reduce sodium? Season foods with herbs and spices. Reduce salt use in cooking and remove the saltshaker from the table. Check labels for hidden sodium. Two slices of white bread could contain more sodium than 1 ounce of potato chips. Look for "no salt added," "low salt," or "no sodium" on labels. Avoid salty snacks, canned soups, condiments, cured meats, and high-sodium processed and convenience foods. The need for salt is learned. If you cut back gradually, you will get used to new flavors and salted foods will taste too salty. Developing less taste for salt is a healthy habit for everyone.

31

OTHER FACTORS THAT AFFECT CALCIUM UTILIZATION

Along with vitamins and minerals, other factors help or hinder utilization of the calcium we consume. For example, dietary fat binds with calcium to form compounds that cannot be absorbed; other substances do likewise. Adding to the difficulty, calcium absorption is impaired in many postmenopausal women and elderly persons. The body can adapt somewhat to low calcium intake or periods of increased need. And one can compensate for factors discussed in this Key: excessive protein intake, certain fiber foods, and lactose intolerance.

Too much of a good thing pretty much describes the American passion for **protein**. It often is heaped so high on our daily plate that it exceeds the **12 to 20 percent recommended portion** of our total food. Too often, it is red meat, sizzling and dripping with saturated fat and cholesterol. Although protein is an essential nutrient that aids calcium absorption, excessive amounts (twice the RDA) promote calcium excretion in urine, washing away benefits. Even moderate increases of dietary protein in perimenopausal women can cause significant calcium loss. The **RDA** is about **46 grams of protein** for the average **woman** and **56 grams** for the average **man** (a chicken breast contains 35 g of protein; 3 ounces of lean beef roast contain 19 g). Purified protein and high-protein weight reduction diets can increase bone resorption enough to cause osteoporosis. Although primarily associated with concentrated protein and not the complex protein found in protein foods, calcium losses can be substantial if a high protein diet continues over a long period.

Years ago it was "roughage" or "bulk." Today this health

98

enhancer that may help eliminate constipation, lower blood pressure, stabilize blood sugar in diabetics, and reduce the risk of cardiovascular disease, bowel cancer, and other colon diseases is called **fiber**. Daily servings from varied foods is best—whole grain breads and cereals, dried peas and beans, and fruits and vegetables, especially those with stalks, skins, and seeds, are high in fiber.

As with protein, there is a hitch. Too much fiber, and components of some fiber, **oxalic and phytic acids**, impede absorption of calcium, zinc, iron, and magnesium by forming insoluble salts. Oxalates are present in only a few foods, among them chard, spinach, beet greens, rhubarb, and cocoa. Recent studies show calcium in the brassica class of vegetables, which include kale, broccoli, and collard and mustard greens, is absorbed very well, whereas calcium in spinach is not. Phytates may be present in legumes and the outer hulls of grains. In amounts normally eaten, oxalates and phytates do not pose a threat if a diet is nutritionally balanced and has sufficient calcium. Absorption of calcium from other foods is not affected when eaten with these components. The average American gets only 15 grams of fiber a day. It is both safe and wise to follow the **RDA of 30 grams of fiber** (do not exceed 35 grams).

Some people have trouble digesting milk *(lactose intolerance)* especially as they get older. This is because they no longer produce enough lactase, an enzyme that breaks down lactose (milk sugar) into a simple sugar, easy to absorb. Undigested, lactose ferments, causing bloating, nausea, abdominal cramping, and diarrhea. Those who suffer distress when they ingest dairy products understandably avoid them, but because dairy products supply most of our calcium, these individuals have a higher incidence of osteoporosis.

Lactose is reduced in some foods by enzyme action or removal processing. Most people who are lactose intolerant can eat yogurt, hard cheese, buttermilk, sour cream, cottage cheese, lactase-treated milk, and lactose-reduced products without difficulty. Look for the words "active cultures," "lactose-reduced," or "acidified" on dairy product labels. Combining small amounts of dairy products with other foods helps slow digestion and often is well tolerated. Helpful products that can be added to milk to break down lactose, and products that release lactase in the stomach when ingested, are available at pharmacies and health food stores. Your doctor or pharmacist can advise you. Individuals who produce very little or no lactase and must eliminate all lactose from their diet must check food labels carefully for hidden lactose in products like salad dressings, luncheon meats, and baked goods, and in medications and vitamins.

Nutrients Pertinent to Osteoporosis Management

Nutrient	RDA	Sources
Vitamin D	400 IU	Fortified milk, dairy products and cereals; eggs, butter, fish liver oils
Phosphorus	800 mg	Beef, poultry, fish, soft drinks, eggs, nuts, dairy products, legumes
Magnesium	300–350 mg	Green leafy vegetables, whole grains, seafood, dried beans, milk, nuts
Zinc	15 mg	Oysters, herring, liver, fish, milk, whole grains
Sodium	1,100–3,300 mg	Processed foods: salt added during food preparation; a natural element in many foods, especially animal foods and dairy products
Fiber	20–30 g	Whole grain breads and cereals, dried peas and beans, fruits and vegetables
Protein	46 g women, 56 g men	Meat, poultry, fish, dairy products, eggs, cheese, whole grains, dried beans, nuts

32

COMPONENTS OF A NUTRITIONALLY BALANCED DIET

Now that we know how dietary factors specifically affect osteoporosis, let's get down to meal planning. Do you recall the basic seven food groups? Foods with similar nutrients are now clustered into just four groups. Less to remember. How nice! Use these guidelines for quick and easy planning of a nutritionally sound diet.

The dairy group: This group includes milk and milk products. They supply protein, vitamins, and minerals, including 80 percent of our RDA of calcium. A serving is 8 ounces of milk. A calcium equivalent is 1 cup of yogurt, 1½ ounces of cheese, or 2 cups of cottage cheese. All contain about 300 mg of calcium.

Include two to four servings daily as follows:

Children under 9 years:	2 to 3 servings
Children 9 to 12 years:	3 or more servings
Teens and young adults:	4 or more servings
Adults:	2 or more servings
Pregnant/lactating women:	4 or more servings
Women over 50 years:	3 or more servings

Proteins: This group provides protein, plus vitamins, iron, and other minerals. A serving is 2 to 3 ounces of cooked meat, poultry, or fish, or 2 eggs. A serving of plant protein includes ¾ cup of cooked dry beans, peas, or lentils; or ¼ cup of nuts, seeds, peanut butter, or tofu (soybean curd). **Two servings daily are recommended.** For less saturated fat, bake and broil rather than fry, serve only lean meat, and choose fish and poultry more often than meat.

Grains: This group, stuffed with fiber, iron, B complex, and other vitamins and minerals, supplies complex carbohydrates, boosts energy, and is an inexpensive source of protein. Foods from this group include breads, cereals, and other grain products. **Eat four or more servings daily.** Because nutrients are removed from grains in the milling process, check labels and *eat only whole grain or enriched products.* A serving is 1 slice of bread or ½ to ¾ cup cooked cereal, rice, or pasta.

The vegetable-fruit group: This group contains vitamins, minerals, and fiber. **Have four or more servings daily.** A serving is ½ to 1 cup of vegetable or fruit. This can be a medium banana, potato, or ½ grapefruit. Eat a citrus or other fruit or vegetable high in vitamin C daily, and a dark green or yellow vegetable for vitamin A at least every other day.

Certain foods are purposely not listed in the four groups. They include candy, desserts, jams, and other sweets; soft drinks and alcoholic beverages; salad dressings, sauces, gravies, and condiments; potato chips and other snacks—foods that add sugar, fat, alcohol, salt, and calories, but little nutritive value. Most of us eat too much of these foods. Include small amounts *only after you have balanced your diet with nutritious choices from the basic four food groups.*

Meal planning can be challenging and fun. Simply choose recommended servings from each group and combine them in creative ways to suit your fancy, your tastebuds, your traditions, and your purse—infinite combinations are possible. Vary colors, textures, and flavors. Not all groups need to be included at each meal, but eating a variety of foods from each group daily will provide a nutritionally balanced diet and help you maintain a reasonable weight.

Serving sizes provide an approximate 1,200 calorie diet. As we get older we experience a redistribution of weight. Our waistline becomes wider. Our metabolism slows and so do we. Less active, we use less energy and need fewer calories. Add hormonal changes, and a woman at menopause may need less than two thirds of the calories she did before to maintain her weight. Individuals who are at a desired weight can simply adjust calories to reduced needs by eating smaller servings and varying food choices. For example, a cup of baby lima beans has 190 calories; a cup of green beans has 45 calories.

Most of us still gain weight as we get older and that may be good. We eliminate a risk factor for osteoporosis (thinness), have reserve stamina in case of illness, have something to fall back on to prevent fractures—literally, extra padding, and with more weight to throw around, we enhance weight-bearing exercise. And wrinkles are less noticeable! However, obesity, defined as 20 percent or more overweight, is a serious health concern. It is a major risk factor in high blood pressure, heart disease, and diabetes and should be addressed with an individually designed, commonsense balanced diet that reduces weight gradually.

Eating habits that begin in childhood are not changed easily. Be patient with yourself. To wean a sweet tooth, serve fresh fruit or sherbet in place of rich desserts. Replace saturated fat and cholesterol with nonfat and polyunsaturated products. Combine vegetable foods for complete proteins. Reduce salt intake. *Read labels and make wise food choices.*

How you plan menus depends on what works best for you. I divide my notepad into sections, label them for a week, fill in menus, and make out a shopping list. Tally calcium and servings from each food group daily (see menus, pages 108–111) to assess your diet, until you have learned the components of a balanced diet and can include adequate amounts without close record keeping.

We each eat about a half ton of food a year; choose it wisely. Use the following guidelines to plan meals for yourself and for your family that will develop good eating habits, improve the status of your bones, and help you grow healthy, and stay healthy.

33

CALCIUM SOURCES: PUTTING THEM ALL TOGETHER

Foods from the dairy group are the best source of dietary calcium. They offer a concentrated supply, contain many additional nutrients, offer economical choices, are convenient to purchase and store, and allow endless combinations for any course or purpose, from breakfast to bedtime, from appetizers to dessert.

Fish canned with bones and tofu processed with calcium sulfate are excellent calcium sources from the protein group. Dark green vegetables, especially spinach, broccoli, chard, kale, collards, and beet and turnip greens, are fairly good sources. Oranges have a small amount of calcium. The grain group has a lot of good nutrients, but little calcium. For the calcium in 3 glasses of milk, we would have to eat 3 cans of sardines, 5 cups of cooked broccoli, 30 eggs, or 18 baking powder biscuits.

Use the four food groups outlined in Key 32 and the calcium values in this Key to plan a diet that will fill your needs, including calcium. Don't get caught up on numbers. After a few weeks you will remember approximate values of calcium-rich foods and can closely estimate your intake as you make choices. Begin with several servings from the milk group. Count the milk in other foods as well as the milk you drink. Use low-fat, skim, and nonfat milk and milk products to wisely reduce unwanted fat and cholesterol. Skimmed evaporated milk and instant nonfat dry milk are easy to store, cost less, and can be substituted wherever milk is used. Responding to a growing demand for low-fat cheese, over 200 varieties are now available. Calcium-fortified foods are becoming more prevalent with raised awareness of osteoporosis. Read labels carefully to be sure that you are getting what you want and need.

Calcium Content Of Foods*

Dairy Group	Food Choices	Calcium, mg
Milk: 1 cup	Whole	291
	Low-fat, 2%	297
	Low-fat, 1%	300
	Skim	302
	Nonfat dry milk, reconstituted	300
	(Powdered: 1 T, 60 mg; 5 T, 300 mg)	300
	Buttermilk	285
	Cocoa, reconstituted with skim milk	392
Cheese: 1 ounce	American, pasteurized process	163
	American, pasteurized process spread	159
	Cheddar	204
	Colby	194
	Cream cheese	23
	Monterey	212
	Mozzarella, part skim	207
	Parmesan, grated (1 T, 69 mg)	390
	Swiss	272
	Cottage cheese, 2% low-fat, 1 c	155
	Ricotta, part skim, 1 c	669
Desserts: 1 cup	Rice pudding, dry mix, prepared with skim milk	277
	Frozen custard, soft serve	236
	Ice cream, hardened (11% fat)	176
	Ice milk, soft serve (3% fat)	274
	Sherbet, (2% fat)	103
	Yogurt: Frozen, nonfat	300
	Plain, nonfat	400
	Fruit flavored, nonfat	300
Protein Group	Sardines, canned, with bones	371
Fish/Seafood:	Salmon, canned, with bones	181
3 ounces	Flounder or sole, baked	13
	Tuna, canned, water-pack	17
	Shrimp, canned	98
Meat: 3 ounces	Beef roast, lean	8

* Data primarily from U.S. Department of Agriculture bulletin, "Nutritive Value of Foods," 1986.

Protein Group	Food Choices	Calcium, mg
	Beef, ground, lean	9
	Ham, canned, baked	6
	Pork chop, baked	4
Poultry	Chicken, ½ breast, boneless, skinless, roasted	13
Egg: 1 large		28
Beans: 1 cup	Soybeans, dry, cooked	131
	Navy beans, dry, cooked	95
Nuts: 1 ounce	Brazil	50
	Almonds	75
Tofu: ½ cup	Processed with calcium sulfate	300
Vegetable-Fruit	Beans, green, frozen, cooked	31
Group: ½ cup	Beet greens, fresh, cooked	82
	Chinese cabbage, fresh, cooked	79
	Broccoli, fresh, cooked	89
	Carrots, frozen, cooked	21
	Celery, 1 large stalk, raw	14
	Chard, cooked	73
	Collards, frozen, chopped, cooked	74
	Kale, frozen, chopped, cooked	90
	Lettuce, iceberg, chopped or shredded	17
	Mustard greens, frozen, cooked	75
	Okra, frozen, cooked	88
	Peas, green, frozen, cooked	19
	Peas, edible pod, cooked	67
	Potato, medium, baked with skin	20
	Potato, boiled	11
	Spinach, fresh, cooked	122
	Summer squash, cooked	49
	Turnip greens, frozen, chopped, cooked	125
Fruit	Apple, medium, unpeeled	10
	Banana, medium	7
	Cantaloupe, ½ melon	29
	Grapefruit, ½ medium	14
	Grapes, 10 seedless	6
	Orange, medium	52
	Peach, fresh	4
	Pear, fresh	19
	Pear, canned, juice pack, ½	7
	Raisins, seedless ¼ c	18

Vegetable-Fruit Group	Food Choices	Calcium, mg
	Rhubarb, cooked, sugar added, ½ c	48
	Strawberries, ½ c fresh	11
	Watermelon, 1 c diced	13
Juice: 1 cup	Orange	22
	Prune	31
	Tomato	22
Grain Group	Bagel	29
	Biscuit, baking powder, from mix	47
	Bread, 1 slice, white, enriched	32
	whole wheat	24
	raisin	25
	French, enriched	39
	Cereal, breakfast, 1 oz, approximately	20
	Crackers, graham, 2	6
	Rye wafers, 2	7
	Saltines, 4	3
	Wheat crackers, 4	3
	Muffins, English, plain, enriched	96
	Bran, commercial mix, egg added	27
	Noodles, egg, ½ c	8
	Oatmeal, 1 packet, fortified	163
	Pancakes, 4", 2	72
	Rice, ½ c	11
	Roll, hamburger	54
	hard	24
	whole wheat, dinner	35
	Tortilla, corn	42
	Waffle, (7") from mix, egg/milk added	179

Miscellaneous Foods

	Chili con carne, canned, with beans, 1 c	82
	Macaroni (enriched) and cheese, 1 c	362
	Pizza, cheese, ⅛ of 15" pie	220
	Soup, 1 c, condensed, prepared with equal volume milk	
	Clam chowder	186
	Cream of mushroom	178
	Vegetable, prepared with water	22
	Sour cream, 1 T	14

Miscellaneous Foods	Food Choices	Calcium, mg
	Salad dressing, ranch-type, low-fat, 1 T	35
	White sauce, made with skim milk, 1 c	302
	Chicken gravy, 1 c canned	48
	Molasses, blackstrap, 1 T	137
	Club soda, 12 oz	18
	Soft drink, cola, 12 oz	6
	Gingerbread, ⅑ of cake	57
	Angelfood cake, ¹⁄₁₂ of cake	44
	Danish pastry, round, with fruit	17
	Sugar cookies, 4, from refrigerated dough	50

Sunday   **Sample Menu 1**

Group	Servings	Breakfast	Lunch	Snack	Dinner	Evening snack
Dairy:	3–4	½	1		1	1
Protein:	2	1	1			
Fruit/		1	1			
Vegetable:	5 or more		2		2	
Grain:	4 or more	2	1	1	2	1

RDA Calcium (1,200–1,500 mg): 1423 mg
(Daily tally for recommended servings per food group and RDA for calcium)

		Calcium mg
Breakfast:	Whole grain cereal, 1 oz (1 c)	20
	Soft cooked egg	28
	Grapefruit half	7
	Bran muffin (commercial mix; substitute milk for water and also add ⅓ c nonfat dry milk)	75
	Skim milk, 4 oz	151
Lunch:	Roasted chicken, 3 oz (½ breast, boneless/skinless)	13
	Potatoes, parsley boiled, 1 medium	11
	Chicken gravy, canned, 2 T	6
	Creamed broccoli, ½ c	139
	Salad:	
	Pear, ½, canned, juice pack	7
	Cottage cheese, ¼ c, low-fat	39
	Whole wheat dinner roll/1 t diet margarine	35
	Skim milk, 4 oz	151

Snack:	Baking powder biscuit/strawberry jam. (Use skim milk for liquid and add ⅓ c nonfat dry milk to batter)	75
	Hot almond herbal tea	0
Dinner:	Bean soup, homemade, 1 c	60
	Saltines, 4	3
	Tossed salad, 1 c (lettuce, tomato, mushrooms, broccoli, spinach) with ranch-type low-fat dressing	70
	Angelfood cake, ¹⁄₁₂ of cake	44
	Ice milk, ½ c, soft serve	137
Evening snack:	Cocoa, 1 c	346
	Graham crackers, 2	6

Monday   Sample Menu 2

Group	Servings	Breakfast	Lunch	Snack	Dinner	Evening snack
Dairy:	3–4	½	1		2	1
Protein:	2				2	
Fruit/		1	1	1		
Vegetable:	5 or more		1		1	
Grain:	4 or more	2	2	1	1	1

RDA Calcium (1,200–1,500 mg): 1508 mg
(Daily tally for recommended servings per food group and RDA for calcium)

		Calcium, mg
Breakfast:	Fresh peach	4
	Oatmeal, 1 packet, fortified	163
	Danish pastry with fruit	17
	Skim milk, 4 oz	151
Lunch:	Vegetable soup, homemade, 1 c	20
	Grilled cheese sandwich (2 slices whole wheat bread, 1 oz low-fat cheddar cheese, 1 t diet margarine)	268
	Fresh fruit salad (grapes, cantaloupe, strawberries), ½ c	18
	Gingerbread, ⅛ of cake	57
	Ice tea with lemon	

Snack:	Fig bars, 4 cookies	40
	Orange juice, 8 oz	22
Dinner:	Fillet of sole with lemon, 6 oz, broiled	26
	Fettucine, ¾ c, tossed with 1 T olive oil,	
	2 T skim milk, 1 T grated parmesan cheese, and	
	dash of lemon, herb, or basil	163
	Collards, ½ c, frozen, steamed, with 1 t diet	
	margarine	178
	Raspberry sherbet (2% fat), ½ c	51
	Club soda, 12 oz	18
Evening	Lemon yogurt, 8 oz	265
snack:	Raisin bread toast, 1 slice /1 t diet margarine	25

Tuesday **Sample Menu 3**

Group	Servings	Breakfast	Lunch	Snack	Dinner	Evening snack
Dairy:	3–4	½	½	½	½	1
Protein:	2		1		1	
Fruit/		1				1
Vegetable:	5 or more		1		2	
Grain:	4 or more	1	1	1	2	1

RDA Calcium (1,200–1,500 mg): 1519 mg
 (Daily tally for recommended servings per food group and RDA for calcium)

		Calcium, mg
Breakfast:	Buttermilk pancakes, 3, homemade, (batter	
	includes 1 egg, 1 c buttermilk, and ⅓ c nonfat	
	dry milk added, yield: 10 4-inch pancakes)	184
	Maple syrup, 1 T	
	Strawberries, ½ c, fresh	11
	Skim milk, 4 oz	151
Lunch:	Tuna, 3 oz, water pack, creamed	92
	Whole wheat toast, 1 slice	32
	Peas and carrots, ½ c	20
	Rice pudding with raisins, ½ c	244
	Coffee, decaffeinated	

Snack:	Skim milk, 6 oz	265
	Sugar cookies, 4, from refrigerated dough	50
Dinner:	Roast beef, 3 oz, lean	8
	Potatoes, scalloped	125
	Green beans, ½ c, with 1 t diet margarine and 1 T toasted almonds	38
	French bread, 1 slice, enriched, with 1 t diet margarine	39
	Apple pie, ⅙ of pie	13
	Ice tea with lemon	
Evening snack:	Banana milkshake (1 banana, ½ c skim milk, ½ c ice cream)	246
	Popcorn, 1 c	1

34

CALCIUM-RICH RECIPES

Remember when staples were butter, sugar, flour, and coffee? Here is a healthier foursome: tofu and nonfat yogurt, buttermilk, and dry milk. Keep them on hand to add calcium power to drinks, snacks, salads, entrees, and desserts. Tofu, yogurt, and buttermilk keep up to ten days and are suitable for most lactose-intolerant people. Keep a canister of dry milk handy to add to soups, gravies, puddings, casseroles, baked goods, cereals—nearly everything!

Fruitelicious Daily Double

2 T frozen pineapple juice
  concentrate
½ c strawberries

½ c skim milk
½ c plain nonfat yogurt
3 ice cubes

Place ingredients in blender, blend until smooth, and enjoy while it's frosty. Substitute any fruit and juice combination; a peach with orange juice is especially good. Yield: 1⅓ c.   **Calcium: 500 mg**

Salmon Almondine

8 oz plain nonfat yogurt
2 T cornstarch
3 T onion, grated or finely chopped
7½ oz salmon, flaked, with bones
  (remove skin)

½ c sliced black olives
1 c colby low-fat cheese, shredded
½ c silvered almonds

Blend yogurt and cornstarch. Add other ingredients, except almonds; mix. Pour into 9" quiche dish. Sprinkle with almonds. Bake at 350°, 30 minutes. Serve with crackers. Yield: 2 c.
          Calcium: 230 mg per 2 oz serving

Vegetable Chowder

1 small onion, diced
1 stalk celery, chopped with leaves
1 T diet margarine

2 c water
2 medium potatoes, sliced
¼ t garlic powder

¼ t paprika
1 c tofu, processed with calcium
1 c nonfat dry milk

1 c broccoli, chopped, cooked
1 can corn (16 oz), with liquid

Saute onion and celery in margarine. Add water, potatoes, and seasonings and cook until soft. Mash tofu and combine with dry milk in blender. Add to potatoes, along with broccoli and corn. Heat over low flame until hot. Serve with sprinkle of celery salt. Yield: 6 servings, 1 c each.

Calcium: 330 mg per serving

Buttermilk Cheese Bread

2 c flour
½ t baking soda
1½ t baking powder
2 t dry mustard
1 t paprika

1 c low-fat cheddar cheese, shredded
2 eggs
1 c buttermilk
¼ c oil

Sift together flour, baking soda, baking powder, and seasonings. Add cheese and mix; set aside. Beat eggs, buttermilk, and oil until well blended; add all at once to flour mixture, and mix just until moist. Pour into greased 9 x 5 x 3-inch bread pan and bake at 375°, 45 minutes or until pick inserted in center comes out clean. Cool 10 minutes. Turn out onto rack. Yield: 1 loaf, 18 slices. **Calcium: 61 mg per slice**

Buttermilk Bonanza

11 oz can mandarin oranges, drained
Mandarin orange juice and water to total 1 c
2 envelopes unflavored gelatin

1 c calcium-fortified orange juice
2 c buttermilk
¼ c sugar or equivalent sugar substitute

Drain oranges. Add water to drained juice to total 1 cup; dissolve gelatin in this liquid over low heat. Mix juice, buttermilk, sugar, and oranges. Add dissolved gelatin. Pour into 1-qt mold. Chill until set. Garnish with fruit for salad, or serve with almond cookies for dessert. Yield: 6 servings.

Calcium: 153 mg per serving

Kale Quiche

2 c skim milk
⅓ c nonfat dry milk
5 eggs
½ c flour
small onion, chopped

¼ t dried marjoram, crushed
½ t black pepper
1 c kale, chopped
1 c shredded low-fat Monterey Jack cheese (4 oz)
½ c parmesan cheese, grated

113

Grease a 10" pie plate or quiche dish. In a blender combine milk, nonfat dry milk, eggs, flour, onion, and seasonings. Blend 15 seconds. Spread kale into dish, pour blender mix over it, and top with cheeses. Bake in a 400° oven, 25 minutes or until a knife inserted near center comes out clean. Let stand to set 5 minutes. Yield: 6 servings.

Calcium: 440 mg per serving

German Cottage Potatoes

4 large potatoes, peeled, cut in ½ inch slices	½ c skim milk
	½ t pepper
1 c low-fat cottage cheese	½ t salt, optional
⅓ c nonfat dry milk	½ t cumin
	½ t paprika

Blend cottage cheese, dry milk, milk, and seasonings in 1½ qt casserole. Add potatoes and mix well. Cover and bake in 350° oven, 30 minutes. Uncover and bake additional 10 minutes or until tender. Sprinkle with paprika. Yield: 5 servings.

Calcium: 137 mg per serving

Double Baked potatoes: Alternate recipe, using similar ingredients. Scrub 4 baking potatoes, pierce to vent air, and bake until tender. Cool just till you can handle them, cut them in half, and carefully scoop out flesh into bowl. Add 1 c low-fat cottage cheese, ⅓ c nonfat dry milk, ¼ cup skim milk, pepper and salt to taste. Beat until fluffy. Scoop potato mixture into skins and sprinkle with paprika. Bake at 400° until lightly browned, about 10 minutes. Yield: 4 servings, 1 potato each.

Calcium: 153 mg per serving

Mashed potatoes: To 4 cooked potatoes, add ⅓ c nonfat dry milk, ¼ c mashed tofu, and ¼ c skim milk. Whip fluffy. Yield: 4 servings.

Calcium: 528 mg per serving

Collard and Cheese Casserole

10 oz frozen collards	½ t black pepper
4 eggs	½ c skim milk
⅓ c flour	1 c lowfat ricotta cheese
½ t baking powder	¾ c low-fat mozzarella cheese, shredded
⅓ c nonfat dry milk	
½ c tofu, processed with calcium	½ c chopped onions

Thaw and drain collards. Beat eggs lightly. Sift together flour, baking powder, and dry milk. Mix with eggs, tofu, and pepper and beat to blend.

114

Add milk, cheese, and onion, and stir. Pour into ungreased 8" x 12" baking dish. Bake 25 minutes at 350°. Cool 5 minutes. Serve with fresh fruit as a snack or entree. Yield: 12 servings, 2" x 4".

Calcium: 206 mg per serving

Orange Yogurt Cake

2¾ c sifted all-purpose flour	3 eggs
2 t baking powder	12 oz plain nonfat yogurt
1 t baking soda	½ t orange flavoring
½ c margarine	1 T grated orange rind
1 c sugar	powdered sugar

Grease 9" springform baking pan with tube center. Sift together flour, baking powder, and baking soda. Beat margarine and sugar in large bowl with electric mixer until light and fluffy. Add eggs, one at a time, beating well after each addition. Add flour mixture alternately with yogurt, beating after each addition until batter is smooth. Mix in flavoring and orange rind. Pour into prepared pan. Bake at 350° for 50 minutes or until pick inserted near center comes out clean. Cool on wire rack 5 minutes; loosen around edges with knife; turn out onto rack to cool. Dust top with powdered sugar. Yield: 12 servings.   **Calcium: 57 mg per serving**

Almond Veggie Stir-Fry

½ c pineapple tidbits, drained	3 T olive oil, divided
¾–1 c pineapple juice	1 lb firm tofu, cut in cubes
¼ T cornstarch	½ c sliced onions
1 carrot, sliced thin	½ c thinly sliced mushrooms
½ c broccoli, flowerettes	½ c green pepper sticks
and stem sticks	½ t coarse ground black pepper
¾ c water	½ c slivered almonds

Drain pineapple. Dissolve cornstarch in juice. Drop carrots and broccoli into boiling water, boil 1 minute, drain. Heat 2 T oil in heavy frying pan or wok. Lightly brown tofu, remove from pan and set aside. Add 1 T oil to frying pan and saute onions till soft. Add mushrooms and green peppers; stir until mushrooms are cooked. Add carrots, broccoli, pineapple, and black pepper. Pour cornstarch/pineapple juice into pan, stir and heat until bubbly. Add tofu and almonds. Serve with rice. Yield: 2 servings.   **Calcium: 333 mg per serving**

Here are other ways to add calcium to your daily diet.

- Buttermilk made from skim milk has only 90 calories per 8-ounce serving. Use it instead of milk in pancakes, biscuits, baked goods—or drink it straight.
- If you have not used tofu, try it. Tofu is soybean protein. Like dry milk, it can be added to many dishes for an economical bonus of calcium and protein. (If you can't find calcium-processed tofu at your local grocery or health food stores, help make it available in your neighborhood. Ask for it, and have your friends do the same. As people embrace more healthy eating habits, the market is responding to a growing demand.)
- Serve the calcium-laden trio—broccoli, collards, and kale— often.
- Substitute milk or part milk when possible in foods that call for water.
- Top salads, casseroles, soups, baked goods, eggs, vegetables, corn chips, and other dishes with low-fat grated cheese; heat to melt when appropriate.
- Add cottage cheese to casseroles, crepes, gelatin desserts, and vegetables.
- Blend 1–2 T of cornstarch with yogurt for a more stable consistency and then use it as a substitute for cream cheese and sour cream, or mix it half and half for more calcium and less saturated fat.

35

BENEFITS OF EXERCISE

Exercise builds bone mass, providing a potent means to stay a step or two ahead of osteoporosis. *And, it's never too late to begin.* The New York Marathon featured three runners over ninety years old; each began to run marathons in his seventies!

The effects of inactivity can ravage all systems of the body. Those who can be active and choose a sedentary lifestyle put themselves in danger. A close look at bones under pressure will expose the critical role of exercise.

Bone mass is built in response to the pressure of weight bearing and the tension of muscles. Bones need this pressure for normal growth and largely become more dense in proportion to the amount they endure. Regular weight-bearing exercise can prevent and somewhat restore bone loss. In a study (Smith et al. 1981), women in their eighties who did chair exercises for 30 minutes, three times a week for three years, showed a 2.29 percent gain in bone mineral content (BMC). A control group had a 3.28 percent loss. Male tennis players (all were over seventy years and had played tennis for 25 to 72 years) showed an average BMC increase of 11.4 percent in their dominant arm (Montoye et al. 1980).

Conversely, lack of exercise fosters demineralization. Bone mass parallels muscle mass. Unused, both begin to waste away, or atrophy. Just as the racket-wielding arm of a tennis player develops stronger and heavier muscles and bones, an arm braced in a cast quickly loses both muscle and bone and becomes thin and weak. Immobility may stem from injury, pain, paralysis, disease, or external restrictions. Whatever the cause, *disuse atrophy* results in osteoporosis.

Were you ever bedridden for a period of time and surprised

at how weak you became? Almost half of our body weight is muscle. If a few months of immobility can reduce muscle mass by 50 percent, it is easy to understand why we becoome weak when we are inactive. Unless there is reason not to, those confined to bed should move their arms and legs, turn, reach, do muscle-setting exercises, or whatever their condition allows, to minimize atrophy.

When a large body area is immobile, perhaps weakened by a stroke, as much as 40 percent of bone throughout the skeleton may be lost. The BMC of three young men, bed bound for 36 weeks, was reduced by 39 percent (Donaldson et al. 1970). Other complications can occur. Calcium leaching rapidly from bones may form kidney stones as excess calcium is excreted, or excess calcium may settle in muscles and joints. Serious problems are likely only in prolonged immobility, in which case precautionary measures are indicated.

Lack of gravity affects bone tissue in a similar way. Astronauts in space for periods of time experienced rapid and profound loss of bone, mineral imbalance in their blood, and increased calcium in their urine. Research conducted in space may help scientists find ways to fight bone loss here on earth.

A type of disuse exists that most of us can control to some degree. A study of healthy young men showed physiologic changes equal to 30 years of aging after just three weeks in bed (DeVries et al. 1982). Half of the slowing of physiologic functions we experience are related to lack of physical activity rather than to the aging process. An effective exercise program can halt, significantly delay, or reverse those changes. Older adults may need to confront loved ones who, in an effort to be helpful, encourage them to "take it easy," or offer "let me do it for you." The very best we can do for those who are able is to let them "do for themselves."

Beyond healthy muscles and bones, enjoy these added benefits of exercise:

- Improved circulation; decreased risk of blood clots and atherosclerosis

- Increased lung capacity; reduced shortness of breath on exertion
- Stronger heart muscle; less risk of cardiovascular disease, diabetes
- Lower blood pressure
- Lower triglycerides and LDL "bad" cholesterol; higher HDL "good" cholesterol
- Improved digestion; bowel regularity
- Improved overall function of all body systems

Regular exercise enables us to put in a good day's activity without undue fatigue and have energy to spare for fun. As we feel better, our self-confidence grows and we are more apt to make other positive lifestyle changes, perhaps even quit smoking. Because exercise burns calories, we can eat more and still lose weight. And we become role models for others.

The argument for exercise is weighted with convincing evidence. The time is right. The fitness craze that began in the 60s and crested in the 70s has become commonplace. Storerooms in office buildings have been converted to work-out areas. Mall doors swing open to welcome early risers who trade window shopping for mall walking, charging their batteries instead of credit cards. Senior citizen centers and retirement complexes have added exercise facilities. Nursing homes are expanding programs as they witness benefits to residents: mobility, mental acuity, self-esteem, and overall quality of life are improved.

Whether prodded by statistics on longevity, moved by massive waves of fitness-conscious baby boomers lapping at their heels, or motivated by commitment to wellness, the fast lane is now crowded with older adults. Wishing to keep their bodies as well-tuned as their automobiles, they are on the move in growing numbers.

36

EXERCISE

No need for the strength of Hulk Hogan, the endurance of Greg LeMond, or the flexibility of Mary Lou Retton. We need only a level of fitness that allows us to live each day to the fullest. Here is basic information we should know, and options that might be fun to explore.

We can engage in three general types of exercise. **Strengthening exercises** build and maintain strong muscles and bones by weight bearing, moving muscle against gravity or resistance. **Flexibility exercises** move joints through their range of motion to keep us limber and mobile. **Cardiorespiratory endurance exercises**, often referred to as aerobics, build overall fitness.

We don't have to sweat a lot to reap the benefits of aerobic exercise. Our heart and lungs can't tell if we are running or dancing; duration and intensity dictate cardiovascular conditioning. Weight-bearing exercises like cycling, skating, cross-country skiing, and running, are great for the heart, lungs, *and* bones.

Intensity of aerobic exercise, gauged by the amount of oxygen needed for the effort put forth, is measured by heart rate. To find your pulse, place two fingers just inside the wrist bone on the thumb side of your opposite hand. Count for ten seconds and multiply by six to obtain the heart rate for one minute. To obtain cardiorespiratory benefit, the heart should work at 60 to 75 percent of its maximum rate, determined by an exercise stress test. To estimate your target heart rate (THR), subtract your age from 220 (your maximum rate), then take 60 percent and 75 percent of that number. If you are sixty years old, 220 minus 60 is 160: 60 percent of 160 is 96; 75 percent of 160 is 120. Your range would be 96 to 120 heartbeats per minute. (Do not use this method if you take medicine to slow your heart.) THR is an average figure. Scaling a flight of stairs might set one person's sixty-year-old heart racing, leaving her breathless, whereas a sixty-year-old friend might easily climb several more flights. Age and condition dictate our efforts. If you have not exercised, are overweight, smoke, or have health problems, your doctor may advise a lower THR, at least to begin. (*Check with your doctor before beginning any exercise program.*)

Base exercise choices on your capabilities and interests, and on social opportunities. Choose what is safe; don't push beyond your limits. Recreational activities are invigorating, stress relieving, and enjoyable, but not always aerobic. However, sports like badminton and tennis can provide aerobic benefits if at least 20 minutes of uninterrupted play occur. Avoid high-impact activities that jar or add undue pressure to weight-bearing joints. Jogging on hard surfaces or horseback riding, for example, may cause microfractures in osteoporotic bones.

Walking is the best exercise of all. It is free, needs no special equipment or site, is unlikely to cause injury, and is most likely to become a healthy lifelong habit. Added benefits are fresh air, sunshine, and time to connect with nature and renew your spirit. Move indoors when the temperature climbs to 80 degrees or humidity to 80 percent, or in cold, windy weather.

Dress appropriately. Cost can exceed cruise fare, but doesn't need to if we skip fashion frills. Loose-fitting garments permit free movement. Shoes are most important. They must fit comfortably and provide good support and cushioning.

Informal exercise in the privacy of your home allows a choice atmosphere. You need only a carpeted area, this book, music, weights, and perhaps a jump rope. Today's jump ropes have ball bearings, require only sure footing and sweep space, and evoke happy childhood memories. You might add a stationary bicycle or rowing machine to your workout area.

Be sure equipment is safe and suitable for *you*. Vary your routine so you don't tire of it. Watch television or read while you bicycle. Use a low-impact exercise videotape. Sometimes television stations show daily exercise programs that you can follow or tape for personal use. Invite family members to share your healthy habit.

Valuing fitness, well-toned seniors are storming health centers, matching younger clients in numbers and dedication. Fitness centers offer many advantages: counseling, education, and monitoring; variety; a psychological boost from camaraderie; motivation through competition; and friendships. Computerized equipment is adjustable to individual needs. Many facilities offer water exercises for those who have arthritic or other conditions that limit land activity. Not all equipment is safe for everyone. Get competent instruction and do the right exercises, the right way.

Private health clubs and public programs and organizations, such as the YWCA, YMCA, local hospitals, community park and recreation departments, and others, offer exercise opportunities. Examine options. Disadvantages may include time and travel inconveniences, or the possibility of being intimidated by the group to exercise beyond your level of safety. Cost may be prohibitive, but it may offer an incentive to those of us who need a reason for regular participation. Not exercising can shorten your life.

Can you substitute daily activities for exercise? They often require great effort. Yard work and gardening are strenuous. Nothing is easy about housekeeping! Your job may be physically demanding. Consider these points: the exercise may not be weight bearing, it may not condition all parts of the body, and it probably is not aerobic. Take advantage of stretching, strengthening, and weight-bearing opportunities as you work and play. Everyday activities are most valuable as a supplement to regular exercise.

37

DESIGNING A PERSONAL EXERCISE PROGRAM

We all occupy a different place on the fitness track. For some, exercise is a way of life. Others never exercise. We are different ages, at different stages of wellness. Osteoporosis may be lurking in the shadows at the turn or already showing its presence by pain and fracture. The same exercise is not for everyone, but *everyone* benefits from responsible exercise. Exercises can be modified, even for those who are bedfast.

From walks in your neighborhood to workouts at a health spa, and everything in between, your program is what *you* make it. To achieve many of the physiological benefits discussed in Key 35, exercise must be aerobic. This Key offers general guidelines for healthy adults. Follow your doctor's advice and adapt them to your circumstances.

Design your personal exercise program

Include exercises for flexibility, strength, and cardiorespiratory endurance arranged in this manner:

- Warm-up: 5 to 15 minutes to gradually raise your heart rate. Do stretching and strengthening exercises, as well as slow walking. Increased blood flow "warms" muscles, making them more pliable and less subject to injury. Include muscle groups you will use during endurance and aerobic exercises.
- Aerobic exercises: 20 to 45 minutes at target heart rate, three or four times a week.
- Cool-down: 5 to 15 minutes to gradually slow the heart rate. Slow walk or march in place; do more stretching to prevent sore muscles. This allows the body to adjust to a reduced blood flow and keeps blood from pooling in leg

veins, causing cramps or lightheadedness. *Never stop vigorous exercise abruptly.*

Exercise need not be boring. Make it fun. Tailor your program to your interests, needs, health circumstances, and lifestyle. Vary aerobic choices. Take a day off to rest. Try weight training, a distinct exercise form that requires professional supervision. Think about these questions as you plan:

- When and where will I exercise?
- Do I prefer to exercise alone or with others? Who will join me?
- Will I need rewards to stay motivated? What will they be?
- What are my time, travel, and cost constraints?

Set goals. If your goal is simply to forestall osteoporosis, walking at any pace can build, maintain, and strengthen bones of the hips, legs, and spine. But if you don't *stop* to enjoy scenery, you can walk at least 20 minutes at target heart rate. Goals should be safely attainable, but also don't underestimate your capabilities.

Walking is an ideal way for a sedentary person to ease into a more vigorous activity. Whatever your program, keep a daily log. It will help you spot problems, evaluate your progress, and make adjustments. It also bestows a feeling of accomplishment, much like crossing off items on a daily "things-to-do" list.

Share your exercise program with your doctor before you begin.

A physical examination, along with stress testing, and gait, balance, and functional range of motion evaluations, may be done to determine what exercises are best for you. Discuss medical restrictions, medications you are taking that might be relevant, and goals. If you already exercise regularly, review your program to note progress and to make any necessary changes. A physical therapist or exercise physiologist may help you design your program and advise you along the way, especially if osteoporosis already is present.

124

Begin your exercise program slowly, build gradually.
Start with low intensity activities. Extend the time, frequency, or intensity as your condition improves. *Include warm-up and cool-down.* Check your pulse at intervals to be sure you stay within your target heart rate. If your heart is beating too fast, slow your pace for a time. Curtail your program if you are short of breath or tired a half hour after your workout. Heart rate should slow during cool-down and approach normal ten minutes after you stop.

Exercise is safe when done correctly, within personal capabilities. Listen to your body. Warnings to stop immediately are pain, breathlessness, nausea, chest pressure, confusion, leg cramps, dizziness, trembling, or a feeling of faintness. You should be able to talk while you exercise without undue breathlessness. Never force movement or exercise beyond the point of pain. Sore, stiff muscles mean they have not been stretched properly, or you have overdone it with exercise that was too fast or too strenuous. Stress fractures and knee problems may accompany high-impact exercise.

Motivation can be a problem, especially before you begin to feel renewal. Exercising with a group or a companion provides support, incentive, and socialization. I walk with my cousin Arleen. We run out of time but never out of conversation, a good lure to walk again the next day. Hold a vision of the benefits: energy, stamina, mobility, independence, and others. Do whatever it takes to continue until regular exercise is as natural as eating. If you reach a plateau, you may seize any excuse to skip a workout. Your routine should be flexible but steadfast. Habits are built by repetition. If you repeatedly miss a workout, that becomes your habit. Be patient. It takes time to undue the damage of a sedentary lifetime. Bone wasn't built in a day.

Be creative. Work out on weekends, during lunch hours, evenings instead of mornings. Reward yourself with an outing. Plan indoor and outdoor exercise so weather is never an excuse. Procrastination is a guilt-maker that can damage self-esteem: "I know I should exercise, but…." Feelings follow actions. Put on your sweatsuit while you procrastinate—then go for it! You'll be glad, once you begin.

Supplement your program with sports and leisure activities.
Square dance for vigorous fun. If you bicycle three times a week and a friend suggests golfing, grab your clubs and go. You may not get an aerobic workout, but you will enjoy fresh air and fellowship, and your bones will benefit from walking. (If you start a new sport, strength training for the specific activity is a wise beginning.)

Incorporate exercise into activities of daily living.
We would hate to give up the labor-saving conveniences that rob us of bone-building exercise. Still, we can greatly enhance the benefits of daily activities if we make fitness a mindset. Unless you will be toting a heavy load, park several blocks from your destination and walk. Use stairs instead of elevators. Even a rocking chair provides more exercise than passive sitting. Rake leaves for compost; string a line overhead, reach high, and hang wash to breeze dry; hoe instead of spraying weeds (a good idea environmentally, too); wash windows with exaggerated gestures and a grand flourish. In fact, do more things with a grand flourish, including living.

Heed principles of back care and good posture.

Evaluate your program at intervals.
It should be dynamic. In a month you may breeze through a routine that leaves you groaning today. Make periodic adjustments.

Your head should be swimming with plans and ideas and your toe tapping behind the starting line. *Ready. Set. Exercise!*

Beginning Walking Program.
Brisk walking burns as many calories as running and is more beneficial overall because one can walk for a longer

Sample Walking Program for Sarah Williams, Age 56. Target Heart Rate: 98–123

Week	Date	Warm-Up Exercises	Slow Walk 5 minutes	Heart Rate	Distance	Heart Rate After 10 Minutes	Walk Time (minutes)	Slow Walk 5 minutes	Cool-Down Exercises	Heart Rate after Cool-Down
1–2	8/23–9/5	X	X	90	¼ mi		5	X	X	80
3–4	9/6–9/19	X	X	84	½ mi	100	10	X	X	78
5–6					¾ mi		15			
7–8					1 mi		20			
9					1¼ mi		25			
10					1½ mi		30			
11					2 mi		40			
12					2 mi		30			
13					3 mi		60			
14					3 mi		45			

period, thus achieving greater cardiovascular endurance and weight-bearing exercise. Walking provides aerobic exercise without a threat to the musculoskeletal system. Adapt this sample to your circumstances. You may not reach your target heart rate (THR) at first. Work up to it and then adjust your pace accordingly. Rest if you get tired. If your heart rate is too high, slow your pace and spend an extra week at that level.

Manage wisely. A realistic goal after a few months is walking 12 to 20 miles a week in three to five sessions at a pace of 3 to 4 miles an hour. Stay within your THR as you make adjustments.

For maximum benefit from your walking workout:
- Maintain good posture.
- Step on your foot from heel to toe, toes pointed straight ahead.
- Move your legs in easy strides.
- Relax and breathe deeply.
- Bend hands, wrists, and elbows slightly and naturally.
- Swing arms freely, rhythmically.
- Smile.

38

EXERCISING FOR FLEXIBILITY AND STRENGTH

If your muscles are rigid and resist bending to your will, they did not become so overnight. Be patient, persistent, and tender.

- Don't bounce or rush; move into position slowly, with steady, controlled movement; hold; release gradually.
- Concentrate on the muscles as you work them.
- Stretch to the point of tension, not to the point of pain. Overstretching muscle fibers triggers a reflex that causes the muscle to contract to protect itself, thereby tensing what you are trying to stretch.
- Breathe deeply, rhythmically; exhale as you tense muscles.
- Maintain good posture.
- Avoid twisting or bending, which puts pressure on the vertebrae and can precipitate crush fractures.

Stretching (Flexibility) Exercises

As your body becomes fit, build to 10 or 15 repetitions of each exercise once or twice a day.

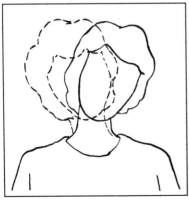

- Head tilt for *neck and upper back* improves range of motion of neck muscles. (Avoid "neck rolls," which can squeeze discs and nerves.) Tilt your head slowly toward the left shoulder, hold for five seconds, then tilt slowly to the right. Do not move your shoulders. Repeat three to five times.

- For *shoulders and upper trunk*, grasp a yardstick above your head. Extend your elbows outward as you slowly lower your hands behind your head. Count five seconds up and five down.

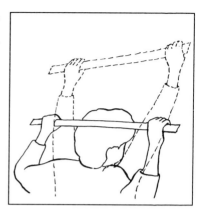

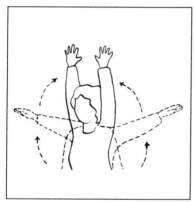

- To loosen *arms, hands, shoulders, and upper trunk*, begin with arms at your sides. Circle them out, up, and stretch over your head to the count of ten. Hold position ten seconds as you stretch your fingers wide for five counts, then make fists for five more. Swing your arms slowly back to starting position. To strengthen *lower legs and ankles*, raise up on your toes while you reach. Repeat three to five times.

- For *shoulders and upper trunk*, hold arms out to the side and make five circles; reverse direction and repeat. Stretch your arms backward, lock your fingers, straighten your elbows, hold the position ten seconds. Slowly extend your arms to the side, then around to the front. Clasp your shoulders with opposite hands. Give yourself a hug. You deserve it! Repeat three to five times.

- The single leg pull is for *lower back, hip, and buttock muscles*. Lie on your back, one leg bent. Bring the bent knee to your chest; grasp it with both hands. Hold five seconds, release, and extend leg to the floor. Repeat with other leg. To add benefits, alternately point your toe

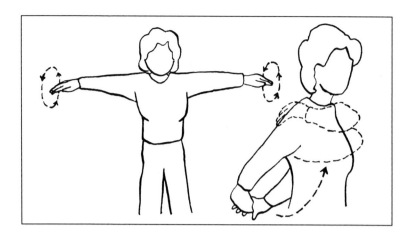

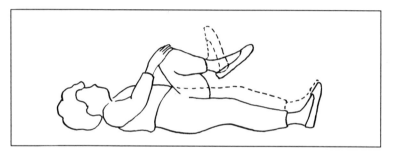

downward and flex it back toward your head each time you
bend your knee. Repeat five to ten times.

- To stretch *muscles in the
back of your legs*, sit on the
floor, left leg extended,
right leg bent, foot against
the left thigh. Slide your
hands down your left leg to
the ankle. If it is not uncomfortable, hold your foot
and gently tilt it toward
your body for ten seconds.
Slowly move your hands

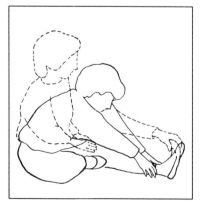

back up your leg. Repeat three to five times for each leg.

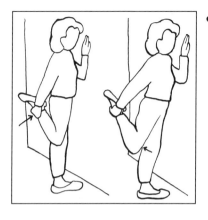

- To stretch *quadriceps and muscles of your knees*, brace yourself against a wall with one hand, grasp your ankle with the opposite hand. Pull your heel toward your buttocks. Extend your leg backward for extra stretch if not uncomfortable. Hold for ten seconds, release. Repeat three to five times for each leg.

- *Calf muscles in lower legs* get a stretch as you brace your head and elbows against the wall, bend your front leg, heel of the back foot on the floor, and lean forward. Hold your position ten seconds, release. Repeat three to five times on each leg.

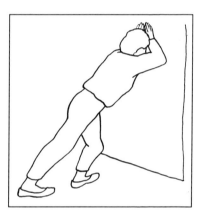

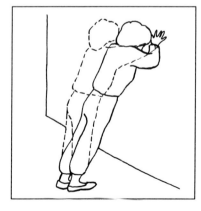

- For *calf and Achilles tendon*, stand about three feet from a wall, hands pressed against it at shoulder height, heels flat on the floor. Keep your spine straight, bend only your elbows, and slowly lean forward until you feel the stretch. Hold ten seconds. Repeat two to five times.

132

Strengthening Exercises

Do these on alternate days, three times a week. (You also can gain strength from endurance exercises, weight lifting, push-ups, and workouts on equipment designed to build strength. Small dumbbells, or 1-pound ankle and wrist weights also can be used. All should be approved first by a doctor or physical therapist.)

- To strengthen *upper arms*, hold 1-pound weights, palms facing upward, arms at your sides. Alternately bend each elbow, raising your arm until it is fully flexed, then slowly extend it back to your side. Repeat eight to ten times for each arm.

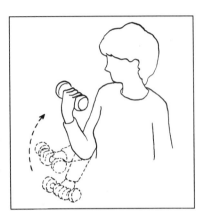

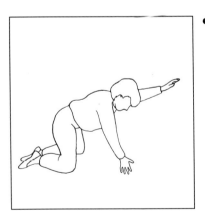

- To strengthen *shoulders and upper back*, get on your hands and knees. With head and spine aligned, right elbow locked, hold your left arm straight out in front, hold for a count of five; switch arms and repeat. Repeat five to eight times for each arm.

- Pelvic tilts strengthen *abdominal muscles*. Lie on your back, knees bent, feet flat on the floor. Tighten the muscles of your stomach and buttocks. Press your lower back against the floor, hold for ten seconds, and release. Repeat five times.

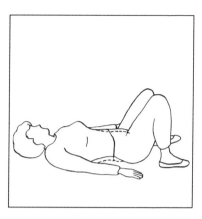

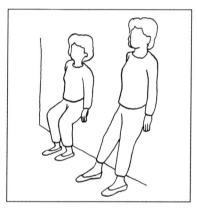

- Wall slides *strengthen hip and thigh muscles*. Stand with your spine flat to the wall, about a foot away, feet slightly apart. Tense your abdominal muscles, and *slowly* slide down to a half-sitting position. Hold ten seconds, then slowly straighten your legs and slide back up, keeping your back flat against the wall. Repeat three to five times.

- To *strengthen hips and thighs*, sit with your legs extended in front of you, lean back, supported by your elbows. Bend one leg. Slowly lift the straight leg as high as the bent knee. Hold five seconds; slowly lower to starting position. To *stretch lower*

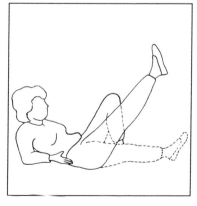

leg muscles, alternately point and flex your foot as you raise and lower your leg. Repeat five times for each leg.

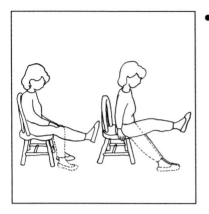

- To *strengthen upper leg muscles*, sit with spine against back of a sturdy chair, feet flat on the floor. Slowly lift foot to straighten knee. To shift the work to hip muscles, slide to the front of the chair and extend both legs, heels touching the floor, hands holding sides of the chair. Lift each leg waist high, then slowly lower it to starting position. Repeat ten times for each leg.

- Strong *back muscles* support bones and improve balance. Lie face down. Keeping your neck aligned with your spine, your hips and abdomen on the floor, press yourself up on your forearms. Hold for 15 seconds. Repeat five times.

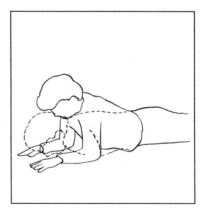

39

PREVENTING FALLS

Natural physiological changes come with age and team with chronic diseases to make us more susceptible to falls. Even minor falls result in broken bones when osteoporosis is present; complications can be devastating. Look at these staggering statistics:

- Falls are the primary reason for admission of 41 percent of nursing home residents.
- Falls are the leading cause of fatal injuries in persons over age sixty-five.
- Half of all patients hospitalized because of a fall die within a year.
- Over half of falls happen at home, in the bathroom or on stairs.

Most Falls Are Preventable

As researchers extend our life span—some say to 120 years in the next century—the added years are merely the oyster. An active, independent lifestyle, free of serious impairment, is the precious pearl we value and wish to preserve.

The following are common problems that contribute to falls and special precautions that will prevent, correct, or compensate for them.

Visual Changes

It becomes increasingly difficult to focus on objects, adjust to light (glare is especially troublesome), and distinguish colors. Cataracts, macular degeneration, glaucoma, retinopathy, and other conditions cause changes in clarity, depth perception, and peripheral vision that cause us to misjudge the steepness of a stair step, the edge of a curb, or hazards in our path that blend with the flooring. We may stumble and fall. *Older eyes need up to three times more light. Use 100-watt bulbs or add fixtures in areas where you move, work, and play. (Use correct wattage for the fixture.) Have regular eye examinations and surgery as recommended, and wear eyeglasses or contact lenses as needed for maximum correction.*

Hearing Deficits

Half of the 20 million Americans who have hearing problems are over age sixty-five, according to the National Institute on Aging. Our ears not only allow us to receive information that advances safety, but background sounds promote security by improving orientation to our surroundings. *Avoid loud noises on an everyday basis to minimize hearing loss. Have your hearing tested and your ears checked for wax buildup. Wear a hearing aid if you need to.*

Reflexes

A reflex is an automatic or involuntary response to a stimulus. As we get older, we fail to react as quickly to hazards or to catch ourselves if we trip or lose our balance. Because aging affects speed, not ability, we still can get the job done if we take more time. *Avoid activities that are timed or require fast action or response. If you drive a vehicle, take a driver's test at intervals.*

Balance and Coordination

Twenty percent of falls occur because we lose our balance. Medical problems, such as inner ear disorders, malnourishment, and thyroid disease, as well as a variety of drugs, can affect the body's sense of balance and position in space. Neuromuscular degeneration, Parkinson's disease, lower extremity impairment, small strokes—even the stiffness from arthritis—can cause an unstable gait. A stooped posture that alters our center of gravity, or a swaying or shuffling gait, combined with slowed reflexes and general muscle weakness, pose a serious threat. *Avoid walking outdoors on wet or icy pavement. Wear low-heeled, nonslip shoes. Plan ahead to avoid a last minute rush. Allow ample time to complete a task. Tell callers to let the phone ring and don't hurry to answer, or get an answering machine. Use a cane or walker if necessary.*

Cardiovascular Disturbances

One fourth of falls are linked to cardiovascular changes. Poor circulation or a sudden change of position that causes a drop in blood pressure (postural hypotension), may cause dizziness, lightheadedness, or even fainting. *Change position slowly from lying, to sitting, to standing. Avoid standing in one position for any length of time; move around or walk in place to circulate blood.*

Drugs and Alcohol

Commonly prescribed drugs and alcohol may cause one to become dizzy, lightheaded, weak, drowsy, or confused, and may impair balance, coordination, and judgment. Studies show that individuals who take long-acting tranquilizers, sedatives, narcotics, and antidepressants that remain in the system for 24 hours or more run twice the risk of falling. Diuretics can cause weakness and fatigue by depleting potassium. Antihistamines, corticosteroids, antihypertensives, decongestants, beta blockers, and interacting combinations of drugs also may cause problems. *Limit alcohol, which impairs reflexes, balance, and judgment, even in small amounts. Discuss side effects of drugs you are taking with your doctor. Medications that are troublesome usually can be adjusted without impairing therapeutic effects or replaced with drugs that are less risky but equally effective. (See Key 10 for other precautionary measures.)*

Hypothermia

As we get older, our body does not adjust as readily to temperature changes. Exposure to cold for prolonged periods of time, either outdoors or in a home environment that is kept too cool, may cause our body temperature to drop below normal. This condition is called hypothermia. It can cause a drop in blood pressure, slow breathing, loss of balance and coordination, mental sluggishness, drowsiness, and dizziness, and predispose one to falls. In severe cases, hypothermia can lead to unconsciousness and even death. Other conditions that render elderly persons especially prone to the complications of hypothermia are thinness, a sedentary lifestyle, heart disease, diabetes, excessive alcohol use, and certain drugs. *Dress appropriately for weather conditions. Keep your head covered and avoid exposing skin to the air. Clothing should be layered, warm, and dry. Don't go out alone in cold weather. Wear a sweater during the day, and bundle up warmly at bedtime. Eat a nutritious diet. Avoid excess alcohol. Keep the thermostat at a comfortable temperature; never turn it lower than 65° at night.*

Ironically, some limits are self-imposed by a reluctance to change and make adjustments. If we need a walker and refuse to use it, we handicap ourselves. Sometimes changes are as subtle as the first colors of autumn; we scarcely notice as hearing fades naturally, and may legitimately ignore the problems that result. If we identify and accept diminished abilities, we can minimize the added threat they pose.

The best safeguard from injury is to maintain the highest possible level of wellness and function we personally can achieve. Take advantage of any aids and assistive devices that will help you manage activities of daily living more safely. Eyeglasses, hearing aids, canes, and walkers can be lifesavers, providing support and security. Think about what you're doing, take your time, use common sense, and take necessary precautions to prevent falls.

40

SAFE-PROOFING YOUR ENVIRONMENT

Just as there are ways to "safe-proof" ourselves as much as possible from internal factors that lead to falls, we also must control our external environment, redesigning it for maximum safety. With pen and pad, do a room check. Identify potential hazards that invite injury and note how you will correct them. When the list is complete, begin the process of safe-proofing your surroundings. Some things you can do immediately; pick up scatter rugs, purchase night lights. Some tasks you will need help with. A family member, neighbor, or local carpenter may install handrails. Here are some "fall-prevention" ideas to apply.

Bathroom
- Grab bars in and out of showers and tubs and near toilets
- Slip-resistant strips or mats in the tub and shower
- Shower stools and hand-held shower heads
- Elevated toilet seats

Bedroom
- A telephone and light next to the bed

Stairways and halls
- Firmly attached carpet or rubber strips for sure footing
- Fluorescent tape along the front edge of step
- Banisters or handrails on both sides
- Well-lighted area, free of clutter
- Raised thresholds or irregular areas covered

Floors
- Spills wiped immediately
- Use nonslip floor wax

- Throw rugs secured by nonskid backing or carpet tape (Scatter rugs are the major cause of trips and falls; unattached, they can become lethal "flying" carpets.)
- Carpeting and rugs securely fastened
- Unobstructed traffic patterns; floors free of clutter
- Electrical cords and telephone wires, book racks, low furniture, plants, and other obstacles out of walking areas and pathways

Outdoors
- Cracked and uneven walks repaired
- Sturdy handrails on steps
- Walk areas illuminated with yard lights

Lighting
- Ample light fixtures and wattage for good lighting, without shadows
- Night lights in rooms and hallways; lamps that turn on with a touch (no need to fumble for switches), special sound-activated devices that switch lights on and off at the sound of a clap

Dress for Safety
Wear shoes that fit properly and have low, broad heels and rubber soles. Avoid loose scuffs, which are easy to trip on, or slippers with smooth soles, which are especially hazardous when walking down carpeted stairs. Loose-fitting clothing and long robes may catch on furniture, doorknobs, or cooking utensils. Pants and nightgowns should be short enough so hems and cuffs will not catch on a heel.

Investigate adaptive devices, appliances, and products that promote both function and safety. Look in the yellow pages under "Hospital," "Handicapped," and "Home Health" equipment and supplies. Telephone to locate a convenient showroom, a catalog, and personnel to help you find what you need.

Of course we can't safe-proof the world, not even our small part of it. Be especially careful when you are away from home. Wet, icy, and uneven surfaces, buses, escalators, building accesses, and poorly lighted areas are especially hazardous. Pets are wonderful, but can get underfoot or trip you.

Half of all falls are due to tripping or slipping. Avoid risky actions that might cause bumps, falls, and injuries. Don't carry objects that obstruct a clear view of your pathway; don't climb on chairs to reach high shelves, or stretch beyond your reach so that you are thrown off balance. Stepladders and step stools become hazards as we get older and are best left to younger folk. Short stools with easy grip handles are less risky. Arrange work and storage areas so that items are within easy reach. Revolving shelves and pegboards work well. Gripping devices function like extended arms for high and hard-to-reach places. Use a cart to transfer hot or heavy objects. For some jobs, it's best to find younger hands to help. It is better to pay someone to clean your storm gutters and wash your windows than to pay with your body.

Plan ahead for emergencies. A portable telephone is handy, for example, to take along into the bathroom when you shower, in case you should fall. A fracture that does not receive immediate attention opens the door to serious complications. If you live alone, make arrangements for daily telephone contact with a relative, friend, agency, or local hospital that provides such services. You can purchase monitoring devices to wear that will summon help at the touch of a finger or sound of your distress signal. Check your phone book for references and your Better Business Bureau for reliable sources. Beyond safety, the peace of mind and freedom from fear of falling is worth all the effort and cost involved in safe-proofing your environment.

41

REHABILITATION

Rehabilitation is the sum of all efforts to restore function and achieve the greatest possible degree of health, mobility, independence, productivity, and comfort. Rehabilitation in osteoporosis may range from exercises to restore full function after a fracture, to a treatment program for someone who is confined to a wheelchair. It utilizes whatever resources accomplish this goal. Assistive aids, exercise, diet, education, medicine, and a modified environment are important components. Human resources include doctors, nurses, therapists, dietitians, social workers, health aids, family members, and other enablers.

Rehabilitation is customized to each person's particular problems and circumstances. For example, rehabilitation following a hip fracture is a slow process that begins with bed exercises and progresses through stages of therapy, using such aids as crutches, wheelchairs, walkers, and canes. The primary goal is to restore mobility. The focus is on physical therapy to build strength and endurance; improve balance, coordination, and circulation; and prevent further bone loss, fracture, and deformity. During the first weeks or months, help is needed with personal care, meal preparation, housekeeping, shopping, laundry, transportation, and most activities of daily living. Needs decrease as recovery takes place.

A person also may be incapacited for some time following the fracture of a vertebra. Here the goal is pain relief and a return to normal activity. Those who live alone are especially needy of outside help. The focus is on medication to ease pain and prevent further bone loss, comfort measures, rest, and a calcium-rich diet. A physical therapist will teach proper body mechanics and exercises to strengthen muscles that will protect the spine from further damage.

The goal of rehabilitation for someone who cannot regain skills or no longer is able to perform daily activities is to foster self-sufficiency by learning to compensate for losses. Therapy includes any measures that enable a person to achieve to his or her maximum potential. A sound rehabilitation program will improve physical, mental, and emotional well-being at any stage or area of disablement.

Members of the rehabilitation team are primary sources of education, information, and enablement, and play a pivotal role in recovery. Along with health principles and rehabilitation techniques, they lavish large doses of encouragement designed to get the most mileage from efforts put forth. Family members can observe therapy sessions to learn how to help with care at home. The following resources will help reduce disability to a mimimum and increase capability to the highest degree possible.

Discharge planner: For those who are hospitalized, a discharge planner will assess needs and arrange for prescribed follow-up care and treatment in the home or at a rehabilitation facility.

Rehabilitation center or nursing home: Rehabilitation after hip fracture often is continued, at least temporarily, at a facility where therapy and care is provided. Exercise and therapy also may be continued on an outpatient basis.

Physiatrist: A medical doctor who specializes in physical medicine and directs, manages, teaches, and applies therapy and rehabilitation.

Physical therapists: They assist with the examination, testing, and treatment of physically disabled persons. They use special exercises, pain control modalities, and a variety of other therapeutic techniques.

Occupational therapists: They evaluate functional ability and needs and use purposeful activities and adaptive and assistive aids to maximize function and independence and promote health.

144

Family/friends: It may be possible to stay at the home of someone who is willing to provide temporary care. For those who recuperate in their own homes, family and friends may take turns attending to personal and household needs.

Home health care: Agencies provide professional nursing; physical, occupational, and respiratory therapy; home health aides; homemaking services; dietary, social, and financial counseling; and other services in the home as needed. Services are ordered and directed by a doctor and supervised by a nurse. Look under "Home Health Care Services" in the yellow pages of your telephone book, contact your local or state Office on Aging (look for the "Health and Human Services" entry in the blue pages), or ask for referrals from medical personnel or acquaintances who know particular services that are reliable and trustworthy. Check references and credentials before you allow anyone to come into your home. Home health agencies are accredited by the Joint Commission of Hospitals and Health Organizations. The Better Business Bureau can help in many cases.

Community resources: Community resources include governmental, religious, volunteer, and senior social service organizations, agencies, and programs. The Office on Aging can supply information and referral. Services vary. Usually nursing, therapy, and personal care; home delivered meals; home maintenance or chore service; and transportation for therapy and doctors' appointments and to senior nutrition sites and adult day care are available.

Assistive aids: Helpful devices make it possible to perform tasks despite disability. With your hands on a walker, tote small items in a carpenter's apron or carrying pouch and ease back onto an adjustable seat to rest. Use a reacher to grasp objects without bending or losing your balance. Dressing and personal care items include adaptive clothing; button aid/zipper pulls; dressing sticks used to pull up pants and skirts, remove socks, or put on jackets; and gripping shoe horns that let you pick up, put on, or remove shoes without bending.

145

There are kitchen aids and devices that help at mealtime. Your home will be safer and more convenient with items such as closet/shelf organizers, lazy Susans, and modified door and drawer handles. Book holders and card shufflers enhance leisure time enjoyment. The list of helpful items is extensive. A therapist can suggest those that suit your needs and provide them, or recommend places that sell or rent them. Make sure you know return options if you order from a catalog.

Helping hands are indispensable, but *you* are most important. Participate fully in therapy, then go the second mile. Be creative as you modify your life patterns. Invite a neighbor to tea and have her do a load of laundry during the visit. Unleash untapped resources. Grandchildren *can* do a bit of cleaning. A neighbor boy might be happy to do yard work or run errands for spending money. Stay in charge and by all means stay involved with other people.

Some elderly persons who are recovering from a fracture may be disabled by a fear that they will fall again. They may refuse therapy, shun activity that is therapeutic, even fail to move about inside their home, afraid of further fractures. They need reassurance and encouragement to build self-confidence, calm fears, instill an attitude of hope, a spirit of faith, and an interest in life beyond their disability.

No longer is rehabilitation postponed until a patient is medically stable; it is part of acute medical treatment. No longer is rehabilitation focused on youth, war casualties, and those who need to regain function to be productive in the workplace; it wisely includes *all* disabled adults, even the very old. Most people who sustain a fracture can return to the same, and sometimes better, quality of life due to new knowledge and the application of a healthier lifestyle. Society as a whole benefits when aggressive rehabilitation restores independence. No longer is rehabilitation a separate entity. It has achieved prominence as a vital member of the health care team. We are all beneficiaries.

146

42

PSYCHOSOCIAL CHALLENGES

Problems associated with osteoporosis and other chronic conditions can be classified into three areas, physical, psychological, and social. In focusing attention on prevention and treatment, too often psychosocial health is overlooked. Other Keys have examined physical aspects and interventions that maximize function and independence. This Key will consider psychosocial aspects and strategies that maximize fullness and richness of life.

All three areas intertwine. Physical changes cause emotional distress, which undermines confidence and self-esteem. Anxiety may bring on depression and disrupt sleep. All influence social relationships. Although most difficulties stem from physical problems, psychosocial repercussions can be just as debilitating. You may recognize these feelings:

- Uselessness: unable to shop, perform household or work-related tasks
- Embarrassment: poor body image, clothing fits improperly, abdomen protrudes, posture is stooped, gait is altered
- Frustration and anger: unable to drive an automobile, dance, entertain
- Anxiety and depression: loss of control, confidence, hope
- Fear: of falling, fractures, incapacitation, abandonment, dependency, death
- Alienation: role changes with significant others, isolation, withdrawal, reluctance to accept help or handle public situations

Problems are magnified by chronic illness. Anxiety is heightened; coping abilities are diminished. Use these strategies to promote psychosocial harmony.

Nurture self-esteem: How we manage stress is dictated

147

largely by our self-esteem. Self-image is how we perceive ourselves based on how we look, what we can do, and how others view us. Self-esteem is how we feel about ourselves based on our self-image. Society values youth and self-sufficiency. When age, illness, and physical limitations rob us of our ability to measure up to society's standards, our self-image and self-esteem plummet. If we accept society's skewed values, we cannot measure up.

An anorexic looks in the mirror and sees "fat" where others see thin. You may look in the mirror and see "useless" or even "grotesque," where others see a competent, beautiful mother or friend. If you consider yourself less significant because you no longer can manage previous responsibilities, you may isolate yourself or withdraw from social interaction. If you don't know it already, learn now that your worth is based on *who* you are and not on how you look, or what you can or cannot do.

Surround yourself with positive people who build you up and help you become the best you can be. Don't invite discouragement by focusing on what is no longer possible; create new possibilities. If you no longer can lead the group, you can contribute wisdom and experience, but only if you believe you have something of worth to offer and stay involved.

Be content with who you are. Look beyond abilities and productivity and reach out to the unique personality of others, and others will do the same to you. Seeing yourself only in the mirror of society is living in bondage to its distorted view.

Continue to learn and grow: Motivation plays a key role in learning new skills, enjoying each day, or adjusting to a modified lifestyle. Mental and spiritual growth can thrive in the presence of great physical disability and can overcome major handicaps. Keep an active, open mind, free of mental cobwebs. Read the classics; join a book group. Sing in a choir. Benefit from diverse friendships and fresh insights. Develop new skills to replace those that are diminished by disease. Can you crochet or tutor English? Look for opportunities to teach, especially young people, tapping talents, skills, and experiences of a lifetime to enrich others, and gaining a sense of pride and satisfaction in mutual accomplishment.

Self-improvement should stem from your own desire to learn and grow, encouraged by others, but not driven by others' opinions. Be curious, enthusiastic. It is your sharpened mind and inner growth that is of worth, not what others think. An occupational therapist can suggest outlets, but you take the initiative.

Stay in control: Physical changes may shift the borders of normal and require a new definition of "self." Do what is necessary to maintain the highest level of physical, psychological, and social well-being. Keep a calendar and schedule daily activities. Arrange to get out at least once a week; invite friends and relatives. Know your limits, then live within their outer edge.

Key 40 considered ways to control the environment to promote function and safety. Now consider aesthetics. A few inexpensive changes can create a pleasant, upbeat atmosphere that will improve your mental and emotional health. Raise the shades and let the sun brighten your personal world. Plants bring nature indoors and add vital oxygen to the air. Add splashes of color with pillows and wall hangings. Handcrafted afghans and flower arrangements inspire conversation and a sense of satisfaction. Scents and music set the mood.

Arrange for tasks to get done so they don't pile up and become a source of stress. If help is available from family members, friends, and neighbors, work out a mutually convenient sign-up schedule. Accept help graciously and without guilt. Your needs are legitimate and may involve the services of a home care or community agency (Key 41). Erase fears and frustrations with efficient organization.

Cultivate a positive attitude: Good mental health demands honest acknowledgement of your feelings. If you deny them, they only will resurface in unhealthy ways. Express feelings of sadness and anger, but set a limit of 15 minutes and then get on with the joy of living. Just as one grieves the loss of a loved one in death, so one needs grieving time for the loss of health, financial security, dreams, and independence. But, hope and happiness also must find expression. Manage your circumstances with a sense of humor, not to deny issues that must be dealt with, but to enable you to deal with difficult issues. Humor allows you to see the the lighter side of the ironies of life, to laugh at yourself. A wheelchair can be a handicap or an opportunity to get where you couldn't go without one.

Build a support system: Nurturing people, who share hobbies, joys, and worries, will offer help and guidance and acknowledge your abilities and worth. They foster a sense of belonging, closeness, and security and open doors to life's fullness. Be selective. Disharmony is inevitable in relationships. Everyone needs one truly empathetic confidante to buffer life's stresses and offer a calmer perspective.

A support group extends an invitation to come out of stagnant waters and drink deeply of all that life has to offer, to share with others who have similar dreams dashed and hopes renewed. Together you struggle and survive, laugh and cope; you are not alone. Osteoporosis support groups are springing up across the country. If there is none in your area, contact the National Osteoporosis Foundation (see Resources) and they will help you get one started.

People and resources are available to help you in sensitive, caring, yet empowering ways to build a foundation of high self-esteem, come to terms and accept what cannot be changed, set realistic goals, and view life with a positive attitude (see Resources). Acceptance is not resignation to your circumstances. It is a challenge to redefine *who* you are in order to appreciate yourself and to achieve and maintain that quality of life that rightly belongs to you. Ralph Waldo Emerson said it best, "What lies behind us and what lies before us are tiny matters compared to what lies within us."

43

THE FUTURE

In the 1990s, we will see many improvements in the diagnosis, treatment, and prevention of osteoporosis.

Diagnosis

Researchers have identified several biochemical markers that can determine the rate of bone loss, and hope to provide a noninvasive biochemical test for osteoporosis. More research is needed to determine the reliability of tests based on these markers, how frequently biochemical tests should be administered, and at what points in a person's life testing should occur, among other issues. Such a simple, inexpensive biochemical test could make mass screening for osteoporosis both possible and practical.

Diagnosis through bone measurement technology, which has improved significantly in recent years, will become even more refined and more widely available during the current decade.

Treatment

To make advances in treatment, researchers need to more fully understand what controls bone remodeling and growth. Whereas available treatments successfully *slow* bone loss, therapies are needed that *restore* bone loss. Researchers will achieve a critical breakthrough in treating osteoporosis when they discover therapies that stimulate bone formation.

So far the known agents that stimulate bone growth are experimental or problematic. Sodium fluoride, for instance, has been shown to increase bone mass, but it does not decrease fracture rates.

Scientists believe that growth factors could offer the ideal solution to the problem of increasing bone mass. The trouble with growth factors at this time is that they are not specifically targeted toward the bones. Growth factors may stimulate growth in all tissues, and, if used to treat osteoporosis, may have side effects such as enlarged organs or tumors. Researchers are trying to discover growth factors that induce bone growth only.

A theoretically-sound treatment modality currently being tested is *coherence therapy* or *ADFR*, which imitates the bone remodeling cycle. The initials stand for each phase of a four-part process: an agent is given to a*ctivate* (*A*) remodeling cycles, followed a few days later by a *depressing agent* (*D*) such as calcitonin, which will decrease resorption. Then a *free period* (*F*) takes place so that the formation can proceed. The cycle is then *repeated* (*R*). More research is needed to determine the appropriate dosages and timing for each stage of this process, as well as overall effectiveness.

The bisphosphonates offer the promise of successfully slowing bone loss and in their more potent forms may stimulate bone formation. Nasal calcitonin is now available in Europe and should be approved for use in this country within the next few years. Tamoxifen, an anticancer drug used to prevent a recurrence of breast cancer, currently is the subject of clinical trials because it also is thought to preserve bone mass and protect against heart disease.

Prevention

One of the most important weapons in preventing osteoporosis is education, and it must proceed in several areas. First, physicians must be educated both in medical school and in continuing education programs not to regard osteoporosis as an inevitable effect of aging. Physicians must learn about the risk factors for osteoporosis in order to counsel their patients at all ages about lifestyle adjustments. Well-informed physicians will make earlier diagnoses, enabling patients to begin treatment before substantial bone loss occurs.

The general public must be educated as well. Awareness among middle-aged and older women has been heightened significantly in recent years, but people at all stages in life must become knowledgeable about osteoporosis. The medical community should disseminate information about such topics as achieving peak bone mass in children and young adults, calcium needs during pregnancy and lactation, and the importance throughout life of exercise that protects bones.

Those who suffer from osteoporosis should fully understand their disease in order to prevent its advance. In a recent study of an intensive program to educate osteoporosis patients about the nature of their disease, it was found that increased knowledge resulted in significant improvement in patients' management of the disease, in positive lifestyle alteration, and in reducing depression.

More research into risk factors and lifestyle adaptations also is crucial to the prevention of osteoporosis. We need to learn about the kinds of exercises that are most efficient in preventing bone loss, the causes of falls, the prevention and treatment of fractures, and the optimum nutrition throughout life for keeping bones strong.

Funding and Other Needs

Although the amount of federal money spent on research has increased substantially in the last few years—from $5 million in 1986 to $33 million in 1990—more federal funding is needed for basic research and to find new therapies.

A crucial issue in the 1990s will be in the area of delivery of health care. The incidence of osteoporosis has increased by 15 to 20 percent in each of the last four years. This is because people seek treatment earlier and they live longer. The aging of the population will continue through the 1990s, and when the baby boomers reach old age, the number of osteoporosis cases will skyrocket. In the near future, we will see increasing demand for more ambulatory care facilities to deal with fractures among the elderly, more sites for bone mass measurements and other diagnostic tests, and more doctors trained in bone disease.

We continue to advance against osteoporosis on every front. By the end of the 1990s, we will have a better understanding of bone cells, including bone building and remodeling, and how hormones and local factors affect the complex process. More specific determination of risk factors and the ways to modify their effect, especially regarding the role of diet, exercise, and safety measures, will help direct our path to prevention. Further clinical studies of pharmaceutical agents and therapies that show promise will provide more effective treatments. The benefits gained from ongoing research may enable you to enjoy a successful journey to maturity.

So now you have them—the Keys to Understanding Osteoporosis. Each unlocks a wealth of useful information that offers life-enhancing potential. But you are the real Key to harnessing osteoporosis. You and thousands of others like you who make the effort to learn about this epidemic disease and apply the knowledge to reap the benefits. Share this book with others to help get the message out, especially to the younger generation, regarding prevention and treatment. Join the ground swell of Americans who are working to make osteoporosis as well known as polio—and just as rare.

QUESTIONS AND ANSWERS

When we are young, we question everything. As we get older, we are more selective about the information we seek. When it comes to your health, it is well to draw from childhood habits. Question everything. The more you know about your body, the better able you will be to take good care of it. Note your concerns and insist that your health care professionals address them in a way that you understand and can follow for optimum health. Here are questions others have concerning osteoporosis.

Q. Laura, age fifty-seven: "My grandmother suffered from severe osteoporosis and I am well aware of its crippling effects. I have studied it and I apply all of the necessary preventive measures in my own life, determined it won't happen to me. I have been having low back pain which my doctor says is from osteoarthritis. What is the difference between osteoporosis and osteoarthritis? Will I be crippled like my grandmother?"

A. Osteoporosis is a deterioration of the bone itself; osteoarthritis is a deterioration of the cartilage in joints. As the cartilage breaks down, bony surfaces rub together and cause pain. Bone spurs may develop over time. Osteoarthritis usually is the result of wear and tear on joints, or the aftermath of injury. Although it does not go away, it rarely causes crippling. Appropriate exercise can be a valuable treatment approach. A doctor can prescribe exercise therapy that will strengthen muscles of the back and abdomen, preserve mobility, prevent stiffness, and promote support and comfort. Maintain good posture and body mechanics at all times. If obesity

155

is adding stress to your spine, it is best to bring your weight to within normal limits. Your positive attitude is a valuable safeguard against osteoporosis.

Q. Cathy, age sixty-one: "My mother and sister always have been allergic to milk products. I never had problems before, but now I get stomach cramps when I eat ice cream or pudding. Am I allergic to milk at my age?"

A. Unlike an allergy that occurs when the body builds antibodies in response to an irritating antigen, an intolerance occurs when something is missing. In your case, it is the enzyme lactase. Normally found in the stomach, it helps digest the milk sugar, lactose. Although you have had an adequate supply, as you get older, your body is producing smaller amounts, which is not uncommon. Most people have adequate lactase at birth and later become "lactose intolerant," a condition more prominent among blacks, Orientals, Hispanics, Native Americans, those of Mediterranean descent, and the elderly. Commercial products, such as Lactaid and Lactrase, eliminate distress but are expensive to use on a regular basis. You should be able to eat yogurt, buttermilk, cottage cheese, sour cream, and hard cheese, because the lactose in these products is predigested. You probably can tolerate some milk. Experiment to find your level of tolerance. Try very small portions, either combined in other food or eaten at the same time. Gradually increase the amount until you notice mild symptoms. Once you know your limit, consume that amount often: buttermilk pancakes for breakfast, a half cup of cream soup with lunch, creamed vegetables at dinner. You will be surprised how much calcium you can amass throughout the day.

Q. Tom, age sixty-two: "I remember years ago many children had rickets. Is it true that osteoporosis is the adult version?"

A. No. The "adult version" of rickets is osteomalacia. Rickets is caused by a vitamin D deficiency. Without vitamin D, the body cannot absorb enough calcium from the food we eat. Without minerals to make them strong and hard, the bones in children bend easily under the body's weight and bowed legs, knock-knees, and other deformities develop. Osteomalacia is a similar disease in adults, caused by a severe deficiency of vitamin D, calcium, and phosphorus. Bones formed without sufficient calcium are soft and susceptible to fracture. Rickets was common until scientists discovered the important role of vitamin D in calcium absorption and prescribed cod-liver oil, a rich source. Rickets are rare today, thanks to vitamin D-fortified milk. Osteomalacia now is caused most often by fat malabsorption or kidney malfunction. Treatment is directed at the underlying cause. Both rickets and osteomalacia usually can be cured with adequate amounts of vitamin D and calcium. Supplements may be necessary.

Q. Mary, age sixty-four: "I was always afraid I would get cancer from hormones so I never asked my doctor about taking them. I am active and I feel fine, but I notice I am getting more and more stooped over. If I have osteoporosis, would it do any good to begin to take hormones now?"

A. You are past the age of rapid bone loss when estrogen does the most good, but it still can halt the thinning that continues at a slower pace in later years. You also can benefit from a reduced risk of coronary artery disease. Hormones are now prescribed in small doses that are considered safe. In most cases, the risk of cancer is very small. Be sure to share your concerns with your doctor, who can identify your particular risks. Your posture indicates that you probably have spinal compression fractures that have occurred over a period of time. A bone mass measurement will show how weak your bones are. Based on your medical history, tests, and health status, your doctor will recommend treatment. Together you can decide what is the best course of treatment for *you*. Careful follow-up with regular examinations by your doctor, Pap tests, mammograms, and breast self-examination will ensure early detection of any abnormal condition and should relieve worry regarding cancer.

Q. Carol, age seventy: "Is it true that calcium lowers blood pressure?"

A. Studies reported in *The Journal of Clinical Hypertension* and the *Journal of Hypertension* show that calcium can, indeed, lower blood pressure in certain individuals. The precise action is not yet clear, and the response differs widely from person to person. At least 400 to 500 milligrams of calcum per day must be consumed. One study found that calcium affects the ability of sodium to raise blood pressure. Reducing dietary sodium may reduce blood pressure more effectively if the diet is high in calcium. Research continues, but there is enough evidence gathered to make it a wise step to get enough calcium. It can't hurt, and you may be one of the lucky ones who will benefit from a lower blood pressure.

Q. Carlene, age forty-eight: "I have checked risk factors and I believe I have little to worry about when it comes to osteoporosis. I am a black woman, heavyset, with no history of osteoporosis in my family. I do not smoke or drink, get more exercise than I care about, and take calcium supplements. My menstrual periods are becoming scanty and irregular, yet I am not suffering with any of the symptoms of menopause my friends complain about. Is there any reason for me to take estrogen?"

A. Although you presently have no distressing symptoms of menopause and are at low risk for osteoporosis, you are forgetting about a major benefit of estrogen—to reduce your risk of heart disease. It also is important for you to see a doctor, preferably a gynecologist, at least yearly for a pelvic examination, Pap test, and mammogram. I suggest you make an appointment. Your doctor can explain the risks and benefits of hormone replacement, based on your personal health circumstances.

Q. Myron, age seventy: "I have kept Tums on hand to relieve occasional heartburn for years. When I heard it also was good for my bones, I started taking a tablet at breakfast and dinner because I don't drink much milk. My neighbor has osteoporosis and her doctor told her not to take antacids. Who is right?"

A. You are both right, depending on the type of antacid you are talking about. Aluminum-based antacids interfere with the absorption of calcium from the digestive tract. If they are used frequently, over a period of time, they can cause bone loss. To compound the problem, some of the risk factors for osteoporosis may encourage the use of antacids. For example, alcohol and caffeine interfere with calcium absorption when consumed in excessive amounts. They also tend to irritate the lining of the stomach and may prompt us to reach for an antacid regularly. Someone who has an ulcer or is taking cortisone also might be using antacids to relieve stomach distress. Fortunately, not all antacids contain aluminum. Calcium carbonate antacids, such as Alka-seltzer, Titralac, and Tums, are good for bones. Antacids that contain aluminum include Amphojel, Creamalin, Di-gel, Gelusil, Gaviscon, Maalox, Mylanta, Riopan, and Rolaids. They are safe to use for an occasional upset stomach, but if they are prescribed on a long-term basis, your doctor probably also will prescribe calcium and vitamin D supplements.

Q. Elizabeth, age fifty-six: "I have been taking prednisone for many years to control rheumatoid arthritis and treat flare-ups. I know that it is a potent drug with dangerous

side effects, but I'm not sure I understand why it causes osteoporosis."

A. Prednisone is one of a group of synthetically produced drugs, corticosteroids (commonly called steroids), whose actions are similar to those of hormones produced by the adrenal glands. They all decrease calcium absorption and bone formation and increase calcium excretion and bone loss and thereby can cause osteoporosis when they are taken on a long-term basis. Anyone who is taking steroids must be monitored closely. Your doctor should have stressed preventive measures you should take, such as adequate calcium and vitamin D intake and weight-bearing exercises you can tolerate. Make sure you are taking the lowest effective dose of prednisone, and if you are taking an antacid for the stomach irritation that often accompanies steroid use, it should not be aluminum-based. Bone mass measurements will enable better management of other drugs that your doctor may order to counteract the effects of prednisone.

Q. Erna, age forty-seven: "As I approach menopause, I am reading to find out what to expect. I am impressed with the value of getting enough calcium to ward off osteoporosis. I find that my body's supply is greatly inadequate. I had kidney stones 13 years ago. Is it safe to take a calcium supplement?"

A. Most healthy adults will not develop stones from a calcium-rich diet, but some individuals must be very careful about any sudden increase in calcium in their diet; even the recommended amount can cause stones. As the body tries to get rid of calcium concentrated in the urine, salts crystallize out and may form stones in the kidneys or bladder. This is more apt to occur if vitamin D intake also is excessive. There are precautions one can take. Medication and certain foods that make urine more acid may prevent calcium stones, which are alkaline, from forming. Your doctor may recommend a diet moderately restricted in calcium and phosphorus, along with lots of liquids—at least 10–12 glasses of water daily—to prevent concentration of urine. Avoid caffeine and nicotine, which stimulate calcium excretion. However, not all kidney stones contain calcium, and dietary modifications should not be made without identifying the composition of the kidney stone and finding the underlying cause. Your doctor probably did tests to identify your specific problem and can direct the best course of treatment. Calcium citrate is the supplement that is least likely to lead to the formation of kidney stones. As you can see, this is a complex, individual problem. Only your doctor has the necessary information to advise you about how much or how little calcium to take. I commend you for your efforts to find out about menopause. Unfortunately, most women rely on their doctor to tell them what they need to know. They are unaware of the myriad of changes that take place during this period of hormonal turmoil. You are an excellent example of a growing minority of women who are seeking information that will enable them to take an active and responsible role in their health.

Q. Judy, age forty-two: "My sixteen-year-old daughter has been anorexic/bulimic for over two years. She runs four miles each day, is bone thin, has not had a menstrual period for over a year, and gets angry when I tell her how she is harming her body. She confides in the school nurse, but refuses to see a doctor. She has been treated for a fracture of her foot, but the orthopedic doctor did not deal with her problem. How can I help her?"

A. Until your daughter decides to accept help, or is obligated to, you probably cannot "tell her" anything. Try to build her shattered self-esteem with positive comments. Both her menstrual cycle and bone mass will return to normal once she begins to eat and exercise properly. Treatment for this disease is not simple and requires professional counsel. The school nurse may be willing to act as a conduit to other professional help. If your daughter is having stress fractures it may be possible to appeal to her compulsion to run and convince her, rightly, that she will not be able to do so for long without proper nutrition and reduced exercise. If that is the case, she might be more easily motivated to seek treatment if a coach at her school convinces her. Evidence of low bone mass on a densitometry test might impress her with the gravity of the situation if bone mass is low. Your orthopedic surgeon may have treated the fracture without considering the whole person. A family doctor may be able to treat mild cases, but severe eating disorders may be life threatening and should be treated by a psychiatrist who specializes in this disease. It is painful to stand by and watch your daughter do harm to herself, especially when it appears to be a problem that could be "fixed" easily. Hospitals and clinics often have special services for eating disorders. I would urge you to call and ask for help immediately.

GLOSSARY

Acupuncture a method of relieving pain or altering the function of a system by the insertion of fine, wire-thin needles into the skin at specific points in the body and the application of manual or electric stimulation.

Amenorrhea the absence of menstrual flow at a time in life when it should occur.

Analgesic a drug used to relieve pain.

Anorexia nervosa an eating disorder, primarily among young females, which is characterized by lack of appetite and refusal to eat, and which results in malnutrition.

Biofeedback a process whereby visual or auditory evidence of functions of a person's autonomic (involuntary) nervous system, such as heart rate, blood pressure, skin temperature, and muscle tension, is provided and the individual learns to consciously control these processes that generally are considered involuntary. It may be used to relieve muscle tension and ease pain.

Body mechanics the body movement and muscle function as it relates to posture.

Bone density/bone mass measures of the amount and compactness of bony tissue within a particular skeletal region. The higher the bone mass or density, the greater its strength and the lower the risk of fracture.

Bone remodeling the process by which old bone tissue is broken down and replaced with new bone tissue.

Bone resorption the process by which bone tissue is broken down and removed.

Bone turnover the rate at which old bone is broken down and replaced in the process of remodeling.

163

Bulimia nervosa an eating disorder, particularly among adolescents and young women, characterized by appetite excess and binges of huge quantities of food followed by forced vomiting.

Calcification the hardening of bone tissue due to the build-up of calcium salts.

Callus fresh bone tissue that forms between and around the broken ends of a fractured bone during the healing process.

Climacteric the period during which a woman's ovarian function ceases and the reproductive years end; the "change of life."

Closed reduction replacing or "setting" broken bones in proper alignment for healing without performing surgery.

Collagen the protein portion of the matrix of bone; composes 95 percent of the organic material.

Cortical bone dense compact bone, 70 to 90 percent mineralized, that forms the hard shell outside of the bone.

Disuse atrophy the wasting away of tissue, including bone tissue, due to lack of exercise, mobility, or use.

Endocrine glands those structures in the body that secrete hormones into the bloodstream, which affect the function of special target organs that regulate growth, metabolism, and most other body functions.

Endometrium the mucous membrane that lines the uterus.

Endorphins morphine-like natural painkillers, released from the brain, familiar as the source of euphoria experienced by long-distance runners.

Enzymes proteins, produced by cells, that serve as catalysts for specific biochemical reactions, such as those used in the process of bone resorption.

Fracture a break or crack in a bone.

High-density lipoprotein (HDL) a plasma protein, containing cholesterol and triglycerides, which prevents fatty deposits from accumulating on the walls of arteries and thus helps prevent atherosclerosis associated with heart disease.

Hormones chemical substances produced primarily in the

endocrine glands and carried to target organs to initiate and regulate activity.

Hypnosis a temporary state of intense concentration in which there is a focusing of attention and heightened responsiveness to suggestions and commands.

Kyphosis an abnormal backward curvature of the thoracic spine.

Lordosis an abnormal forward curvature of the lower (lumbar) spine.

Low-density lipoprotein (LDL) a plasma protein, containing large amounts of cholesterol and triglycerides, associated with increased fatty deposits in blood vessels.

Magnetic resonance imaging (MRI) a technique whereby a clear image of the inside of the body is produced through the use of magnetism and radio waves. A computer translates the pattern of magnetic energy into an image.

Matrix the protein network of bone in which minerals are deposited.

Menarche the first menstrual period and the beginning of menstruation, usually between ages nine and seventeen.

Menopause the final menstrual period. The term is commonly used to describe the entire period of diminishing ovarian function.

Metabolism the process by which the body converts food into energy and living tissue.

Mineralization the addition of minerals, mainly calcium and phosphorus, to bone in the process of building bone tissue.

Narcotic a drug that in moderate doses depresses the central nervous system, relieves pain, and produces sleep, and in excessive doses produces unconsciousness, stupor, coma, and possibly death.

Necrosis death of areas of tissue contained within healthy tissue.

Nutrients food or liquid that promotes life by providing nourishment for growth, repair, and metabolism of body tissues.

165

Open reduction a surgical procedure by which an incision is made and parts of a fractured bone are set into proper position and fixed in place with hardware.

Ossification the formation of true bone from cartilage or fibrous tissue in early life or from the clot that forms after a fracture.

Osteoblasts cells located in the periosteum, responsible for bone-building and repair.

Osteoclasts cells that secrete enzymes and acids that dissolve bone cells, creating minute holes in bone, suitable for deposit of new tissue by osteoblasts.

Osteocytes cells embedded in the matrix of mineralized bone. They are osteoblasts that have completed their initial function to build bone tissue and then become maintenance cells, transmitting information and helping in the exchange of calcium salts between bone and bloodstream.

Osteomalacia the softening of bones in adults due to impaired mineralization, which results from a vitamin D deficiency.

Osteoporosis a disease characterized by low bone mass, microarchitectural deterioration of bone tissue leading to enhanced bone fragility, and a consequent increase in fracture risk.

Ovulation the discharge of the ovum (egg) from the graafian follicle of the ovary.

Perimenopausal the period of diminishing ovarian function during which the body prepares for menopause.

Periosteum the fibrous membrane that covers bone, except at the joints.

Posture an attitude or position of the body.

Puberty the age when the reproductive organs begin to function.

Recommended Dietary Allowances (RDAs) guidelines for all age levels for the amounts of particular nutrients needed on a daily basis to maintain health and keep the normal population well nourished.

Rehabilitation the treatment and education that leads to the restoration of a person to a former state of health or to the attainment of maximum function and well-being.

Rickets a condition of the young caused by a deficiency of vitamin D, which leads to altered calcium and phosphorus metabolism and consequent disturbance of bone formation.

Risk factors factors that predispose an individual to the development of a disease or condition.

Screening mass testing of populations for a disease or condition so that action can be taken before it worsens. Selective screening involves testing those populations who are at greater risk.

Trabecular bone the honeycombed inner bone, encased within an outer shell of cortical bone, nourished by the marrow that fills its hollow cavities.

Traction tension or force exerted on bone or body part to correct malformation, maintain proper position, and aid healing in treating certain fractures.

Vertebra any one of the small bony segments of the spine.

RESOURCES

Organizations

American Association of Retired Persons (AARP) Materials include: *Pep Up Your Life* (D549), exercises for people over 50; *Eating for Your Health* (D12164), a guide to special diets; *Action for a Healthier Life* (D13474): A guide for Midlife and Older Women; *Healthy Questions* (D12094), selecting health professionals; and *Chances Are You Need a Mammogram* (D14502); discusses benefits of mammography screening for women 50 and over. For a free copy, send the title(s) and stock number(s) on a postcard to: AARP Fulfillment (EE0231) 601 E. Street, N.W., Washington, D.C. 20049.

American Physical Therapy Association (APTA) Brochures include: *The Secret of Good Posture*, *Taking Care of Your Back*, and *Fitness: A Way of Life*. APTA, 1111 North Fairfax Street, Alexandria, Virginia 22314.

Consumer Information Center, Pueblo, Colorado 81009. Booklets free or at minimal charge on a large variety of topics: food, health, safety, fitness, exercise, travel, how to access government agencies for help, who to contact and how, and more. *Consumer Information Catalog* and *Consumer's Resource Handbook* list resources.

Food and Drug Administration (FDA) Consumer Inquiries Staff. HFE-88, 5600 Fishers Lane, Rockville, Maryland 20857. (301) 443-3170. (Local FDA office is listed in phone books under U. S. Health and Human Services.) Free informational brochures and answers to questions on FDA-regulated items: drugs, food, labeling, and more.

National Dairy Council, 6300 North River Road, Rosemont, Illinois 60018-4233. (708) 696-1860. Brochures, most are free, include: *Osteoporosis: Are You At Risk?, All-American Guide to Calcium-Rich Foods, Getting Along with Milk: For People with Lactose Intolerance, Calcium: You Never Outgrow Your Need for It, Every Woman's Guide to Health and Nutrition*, plus fact sheets on milk, cheese, cultured products, yogurt, butter, ice cream, basic four food groups, and a catalog.

National Institute on Aging (NIA) Free materials include: *Preventing Falls and Fractures, Accidents and the Elderly, Dietary Supplements: More is Not Always Better, Be Sensible About Salt, Safe Use of Medicines by Older People, Health Resources for Older Women, Don't Take it Easy—Exercise!, Exercise Program Packet*, and *The Menopause Time of Life*, a booklet about changes, surgical menopause, hormone replacement, emotions, and sexuality. NIA Information Center/ Pl, 2209 Distribution Circle, Silver Spring, Maryland 20910. (301) 495-3455.

National Osteoporosis Foundation (NOF) This nonprofit organization provides research support, advocates for federal support, and works with organizations, federal agencies, medical institutions and personnel, and the public to educate consumers and health care professionals about osteoporosis. Annual membership dues of $25 (individual) and $10 (retiree), include subscription to *The Osteoporosis Report* newsletter, *Boning up on Osteoporosis* booklet, legislative and medical updates, and discounts on NOF materials. NOF encourages support groups and will direct you to one in your area or help you get one started. National Osteoporosis Foundation, 2100 M Street, N.W., Suite 602, Washington D.C. 20037.

Public and medical libraries and organizations and agencies, such as the American Heart Association, Arthritis Association, and Office on Aging, can provide information and direction. Many hospitals offer programs, educational materials, support groups, and professionals who supply health-related information. Senior citizen centers and community and religious groups may fill psychosocial needs.

Books, Catalogs, Pamphlets, and Tapes

A Cheese Lover's Guide to Lower Fat Cheeses Lists calorie, cholesterol, fat, and calcium content of types and brands of cheese. Send self-addressed, stamped business envelope and $1 to Dairy Council of Wisconsin, Inc., Westmont, Illinois 60559.

Aids for Arthritis—Self-Help Products Catalog of aids and appliances for handicapped persons. Aids for Arthritis, 3 Little Knoll Ct., Medford, New Jersey 08055.

Boning Up on Osteoporosis Booklet on causes, prevention, and treatment of osteoporosis. Send check for $1.75 to the National Osteoporosis Foundation, 2100 M Street, N.W., Suite 602, Washington, D.C. 20037.

*Calcium and Common Sense Heaney, Robert P., and M. Janet Barger-Lux. New York: Doubleday, 1988. (Available at public libraries.)

*Calcium: How Important Is It? Free pamphlet of information on calcium use in the body and on osteoporosis prevention, along with high-calcium menus and recipes. Giant Food, Inc., P.O. Box 1804, Washington, D.C. 20013. (301) 341-4100.

* This work was aided in part by the National Arthritis and Musculoskeletal and Skin Diseases Information Clearinghouse.

Fitness Fundamentals Personal exercise booklet with fitness information for various groups, including the elderly (no. 017-001-00453-7). *Walking for Exercise and Pleasure.* 12-page brochure, $1 (no. 017-00100447-2). President's Council on Physical Fitness and Sports. Superintendent of Documents, U.S. Government Printing Office, Washington, D.C. 20402.

Home Health Care Resource Catalog Clothing, equipment, and supplies for persons with disabilities. Free at local Sears, Roebuck and Co. stores.

Living With Chronic Illness: Days of Patience and Passion Register, Cheri. New York: Bantam, 1987. (Available at public libraries.)

Nutritive Value of Foods Commonly used foods and RDAs. Human Nutrition Information Service, U. S. Department of Agriculture Home and Garden, bulletin no. 72, $3, from the Superintendent of Documents, U.S. Government Printing Office, Washington, D.C. 20401, or any U.S. Government Printing Office bookstore.

Osteoporosis: Cause, Treatment, Prevention 38 pages. Send business-size self-addressed envelope stamped with 2 first-class U.S. postage stamps to Osteoporosis Booklet, National Institutes of Health, Box AMS, Bethesda, Maryland 20892. (301) 468-3235.

Smith & Nephew Rolyan. Daily living products; 40-page catalog of dressing, hygiene, and homemaking aids, wheelchair accessories, and more. 1-800-558-8633.

Stretching Bob Anderson. Exercises designed to promote lifelong flexibility and movement. Shelter Publishers, 1980. (Available at public libraries.)

Swing Into Shape Three 30-minute videos of low-intensity workouts. Exercises at different levels of intensity, done from sitting and standing positions. Focus is on stretching, toning, and endurance strengthening. Cost, $39.95 or $14.95 per video plus shipping and handling. Lutheran Hospital, Department of Education, 1910 South Ave., La Crosse, Wisconsin 54601. (608) 785-0530, ext. 3194.

We Are Not Alone: Learning to Live With Chronic Illness Pitzele, Sefra Kobrin. New York: Workman, 1986. (Available at public libraries.)

The Calcium Bible Hausman, Patricia. New York: Rawson, 1985. Contains information regarding the role of calcium through ages and stages of life and special diets and health problems; a calcium counter; recipes; provides a means to evaluate your personal calcium needs and intake. (Available at public libraries.)

The Strong Bones Diet Goulder, Lois, and Leo Lutwak. Gainsville, Florida: Triad, 1988. Information on nutrition, and recipes that promote bone health. (Available at public libraries.)

BIBLIOGRAPHY

Beland, Irene L., and Joyce Y. Passos. *Clinical Nursing: Pathophysiological and Psychosocial Approaches.* 4th ed. New York: Macmillan, 1981.

Berkow, Robert, ed. *Merck Manual of Diagnosis and Therapy.* 15th ed. Rahway, New Jersey: Merck Sharp & Dohme, 1987.

Berstein, Ellen, ed. *Medical and Health Encyclopedia Brittanica.* Chicago, 1991.

Burnside, Irene. *Nursing and the Aged: A Self-Care Approach.* 3d ed. New York: McGraw-Hill, 1988.

Calcium: A Summary of Current Research for the Health Professional. National Dairy Council. 2d ed. 1989.

Carnevali, Doris L., and Maxine Patrick, eds. *Nursing Management For The Elderly*, 2d ed. New York: Lippincott, 1986.

Chestnut, Charles H., III. "Osteoporosis and Its Treatment." *New England Journal of Medicine.* February 6, 1992, p. 406–7. Editorial comment.

Clayman, Charles B., ed. *The American Medical Association Guide to Prescription and Over-the-Counter Drugs.* New York: Random House, 1988.

Cummings, Steven R., et. al. "Should Prescription of Post-menopausal Hormone Therapy be Based on the Results of Bone Densitometry?" Editorial comment. *Annals of Internal Medicine.* 113; 8 (1990): 565–6.

Dalsky, Gail P., et. al. "Weight-Bearing Exercise Training and Lumbar Bone Mineral Content in Postmenopausal Women." *Annals of Internal Medicine.* 108 (1988): 824–8.

DeVries, Herbert A., et. al. "Exercise: Getting the elderly going." *Client Care*, October 15, 1982: 67–111.

Dhuper, S., et. al. "Effects of hormonal status on bone density in adolescent girls." *Journal of Clinical Endocrinology and Metabolism.* 71; 5 (1990): 1083–8.

Donaldson, Charles L., et. al. "Effect of prolonged bedrest on bone mineral." *Metabolism.* 19 (1970): 1071–84.

Drinkwater, Barbara L. "Physical exercise and bone health." *Journal of the American Medical Women's Association.* 45; 3 (1990): 91–7.

Ebersole, Pricilla, and Patricia Hess. *Toward Healthy Aging: Human Needs and Nursing Response.* 3d ed. St. Louis: Mosby, 1990.

Eschleman, Marian Maltese. *Introductory Nutrition and Diet Therapy.* Philadelphia: Lippincott, 1984.

Ferrell, Betty R., and Bruce A. "Easing the PAIN." *Geriatric Nursing.* (Jul/Aug 1990): 175–8.

Ferrini, Armeda F., and Rebecca L. *Health in the Later Years.* Dubuque: Brown, 1989.

Garland, Cedric, et. al. *The Calcium Connection.* New York: Simon & Schuster, 1989.

Gates, Sharon J., ed and Pekka A. Mooar. *Orthopaedics and Sports Medicine for Nurses.* Baltimore: Williams & Wilkins, 1989.

Gebhardt, Susan E., and Ruth H. Mathews. U.S. Department of Agriculture, Human Nutrition Information Service. *Nutritive Value of Foods.* Home and Garden bulletin no. 72, 1986.

Gluer, Claus C., et. al. "Comparative Assessment of Dual-Photon Absorptiometry and Dual-Energy Radiography." *Radiology.* 174(1990): 223-8.

Grisso, Jean A., et. al. "Risk Factors for Falls as a Cause of Hip Fractures in Women." *New England Journal of Medicine.* 324; 19 (1991): 1326–1330.

Heany, Robert P., "Calcium intake in the osteoporotic fracture context: introduction." *American Journal of Clinical Nutrition.* 54 (1991): 242S–244S.

——. "Calcium intake and bone health throughout life."

Journal of the American Medical Women's Association.
45; 3 (1990): 80–6.

Heany, Robert P., and Connie M. Weaver. "Calcium absorption of kale." *American Journal of Clinical Nutrition.* 51 (1990): 656–7.

Huddleston, Alan L., et. al. "Bone Mass in Lifetime Tennis Players." *Journal of the American Medical Association.* 244 (1980): 1107–9.

Jackson, Jeffrey A., and Michael Kleerekoper. "Osteoporosis in Men: Diagnosis, Pathophysiology, and Prevention," *Medicine.* 69; 3 (1990): 137–152.

Johnston, C. Conrad, Jr., and Christopher Longcope. "Premenopausal Bone Loss—A Risk Factor for Osteoporosis." *New England Journal of Medicine.* 323: 18 (1990): 1271–2.

Larson, David E., ed. *Mayo Clinic Family Health Book.* New York: Morrow, 1990.

Licata, Angelo A. "Therapies for symptomatic primary osteoporosis." *Geriatrics.* 46; 11 (1991): 62–7.

Loebl, Suzanne, et. al. *The Nurses' Drug Handbook.* 6th ed. Albany: Delmar, 1991.

Maas, Meridean, Kathleen C. Buckwalter, and Mary Hardy. *Nursing Diagnosis and Interventions for the Elderly.* New York: Addison-Wesley, 1991.

Mazess, Richard B., et. al. "Skeletal and body-composition effects of anorexia nervosa." *American Journal of Clinical Nutrition.* 52 (1990): 438–441.

McKenry, Leda M., and Evelyn Salerno. *Pharmacology in Nursing.* 17th ed. Philadephia: Mosby, 1989.

McKeon, Valerie Ann. "Estrogen Replacement Therapy." *Journal of Gerontological Nursing.* 16; 10 (1990): 6–11.

Meuleman, John. "Osteoporosis and the Elderly." *Medical Clinic of North America.* 73; 6 (1989): 1455–70.

Miller, Carol A. *Nursing Care of Older Adults: Theory and Practice.* Glenview, Illinois: Scott, Foresman, 1990.

Montoye, Henry J., et. al. "Bone mineral in senior tennis

players." *Scandinavian Journal of Sports and Science.* 2 (1990): 26–32.

Morgan, Brian L.G., and Roberta. *Hormones: how they affect behavior, metabolism, growth, development and relationships.* Los Angeles: Body Press-Price, 1989.

Osteoporosis: Current Concepts. Report of the Seventh Ross Conference on Medical Research. Columbus: Ross, 1987.

Peck, William A. "Estrogen therapy (ET) after menopause." *Journal of the American Medical Women's Association.* 45; 3 (1990): 87–90.

Riggs, B. Lawrence, and L. Jospeh Melton III. "Involutional Osteoporosis." *New England Journal of Medicine.* 314 (1986): 1676–86.

———. "Clinical Heterogeneity of Involutional Osteoporosis: Implications for Preventive Therapy." *Journal of Clinical Endocrinology and Metabolism.* 70; 5 (1990): 1229–32.

Roberto, Karen A. "Women with Osteoporosis: The Role of the Family and Service Community." *The Gerontologist.* 28; 2 (1988): 224–228.

Smith Everett L. Jr., et. al. "Physical activity and calcium modalities for bone mineral increase in aged women." *Medicine and Science in Sports and Exercise.* 13 (1981): 60–4.

Stampfer, Mier J., et. al. "Postmenopausal Estrogen Therapy and Cardiovascular Disease." *New England Journal of Medicine.* 325; 11 (1991): 756–61.

Tinnetti, Mary E. "Fall Risk Index for Elderly patients Based on Number of Chronic Disabilities. *American Journal of Medicine.* 80 (1986): 429–34.

Tollison, C. David, and Michael L. Kriegel. "Bone Loss and Physical Inactivity: Can Exercise Prevent Osteoporosis?" *Journal of the South Carolina Medical Association.* (March 1990): 138–140.

Tosteson, Anna N.A., et. al. "Cost Effectiveness of Screening Perimenopausal White Women for Osteoporosis: Bone Densitometry and Hormone Replacement Therapy."

Annals of Internal Medicine. 113; 8 (1990); 594–603.

Treatments. Nurses Reference Library. Springhouse, Pennsylvania. Nursing '88 Books.

United States Pharmacopeia: Drug Information for the Consumer. Mount Vernon, New York: Consumers Union, 1989.

U.S. Department of Health and Human Services. *Osteoporosis Research, Education and Health Promotion.* National Institutes of Health, 1991.

Wahner, Heinz W. et. al. "Comparison of Dual-Energy X-Ray Absorptiometry and Dual Photon Absorptiometry for Bone Mineral Measurements of the Lumbar Spine." *Mayo Clinic Proceedings.* 63 (1988): 1075–84.

Wasnich, Richard D., et. al. "Appropriate clinical application of bone density measurements." *Journal of the American Medical Women's Association.* 45 (1990): 99–102.

Watts, Nelson B., et. al. "Intermittent Cyclical Etidronate Treatment of Postmenopausal Osteoporosis." *New England Journal of Medicine.* 323; 2 (1990): 74–9.

Webster, JoAnne A. "Key to Healthy Aging: Exercise." *Journal of Gerontological Nursing.* 14; 12 (1988): 9–15.

Witte, Melanie. "Pain Control." *Journal of Gerontological Nursing.* 15; 3 (1989): 32–7.

World Book Encyclopedia. Chicago: Scott-Fetzer, 1991.

INDEX

Gonads, 11
Grains, 102
Growth factors, 151–152
Growth hormones (GH), 10, 12
Gynecologist, 36

Hallway safety, 140
Hearing deficits, 137
Heat, 61–62
High-density lipoprotein (HDL), 89
Hip fractures, 2, 48–50
Home health care, 145
Hormone Replacement Therapy (HRT), 22, 23, 71–73
Hormones, 10–12
  imbalance of, 24–25
Hyperparathyroidism, 24–25
Hypnosis, 64
Hypothermia, 138–139

Ibuprofen, 59
Idiopathic osteoporosis, 33
Imagery, 64
Insulin, 25

Juvenile osteoporosis, 33

Kyphosis (dowager's hump), 18, 20, 53, 54
Lactose intolerance, 99–100
Laughter, 65
Lifting, 79

Lighting for safety, 141
Lordosis, 53
Low-density lipoprotein (LDL), 89
Luteinizing hormones (LH), 10
Lying/sleeping, 80

Magnesium, 96–97
Magnetic resonance imaging (MRI), 41, 47
Management program, 82–83
Matrix (bone), 7–9
Medication
  analgesics, 57–59
  management of, 29
Meditation, 64
Medulla, 11
Men, 31–32
Menarche, 21
Menopause, 22
Menus, calcium-rich, 108–111
Meperidine, 58
Metabolism, 6, 90
Milk, 91
Mineralization, 5
Minerals, 90
Morphine, 58

National Dairy Council, 169
National Institute on Aging, 169
National Osteoporosis Foundation, 43, 81, 169

Neutron activation, 37
Nonsteroidal anti-inflammatory drugs (NSAIDS), 58, 59
Nursing home, 144
Nutrients:
  carbohydrates, 88–89
  fats, 89
  for osteoporosis management, 100
  proteins, 89
  vitamins and minerals, 90
  water, 90
Nutrition, 81
  basic, 88–90

Obesity, 103
Occupational therapist, 56, 144
Open reduction, 45, 46
Organizations, 168–170
Orthopedist, 37
Ossification, 46
Osteoblasts, 8–9
Osteoclasts, 8, 10–11, 24
Osteocytes, 9
Osteogenesis imperfecta, 33
Osteomalacia, 95
Osteoporosis
  advanced, management program for, 84–87
  definition of, 1
  drugs causing, 27–30
  future diagnosis, treatment, and prevention of, 151–154

men and, 31–32
nutrients for management of, 100
postmenopausal, 21–23
risk factors for, 13–17, 81
secondary causes of, 24–26
senile, 18–20
youth and, 33–35
Outdoor safety, 141
Ovaries, 11, 23
Overexercise, 26
Ovulation, 21
Oxalic acid, 99

Pain
  acute, 57
  chronic, 57
  gate theory and, 60
  measures for alleviating, 60–62
  relaxation techniques for, 63–65
Pamphlets, 170–172
Parathormone (PTH), 10–11, 19, 76
Parathyroid glands, 10–11
Perimenopausal years, 22
Periosteum, 6
Phenytoin (Dilantin), 28
Phosphorus, 96
Physiatrist, 37, 144
Physical therapist, 56, 144
Phytic acid, 99
Pituitary gland, 10
Positive attitude, 149–150

Testosterone, 11, 31–32
Tests, medical, 37–38
Tetracycline, 28
Therapeutic touch, 64
Thyroid gland, 11
Thyroid stimulating
    hormones (TSH), 10
Thyroid supplements, 28
Thyroxine, 11
Trabecular bone, 6, 18–19,
    22
Traction, 45, 46
Transcutaneous electrical
    nerve stimulation
    (TENS), 60–61
Treatment, 151–152
Triiodothyronine, 11

Ultrasound, 41, 62

Unsaturated fats, 89
Urine test, 38

Vegetable-fruit group, 102
Vertebrae, 53
Vesalius, Andreas, 4
Visual changes, 136–137
Vitamin D, 19, 76, 95–96
Vitamins, 90

Walking program, 126–128
Warm-up exercises, 123
Water, 90
Weight gain, 103
Wrist fracture, 50–51

X ray, 37

Zinc, 97